1,000,000 Books

are available to read at

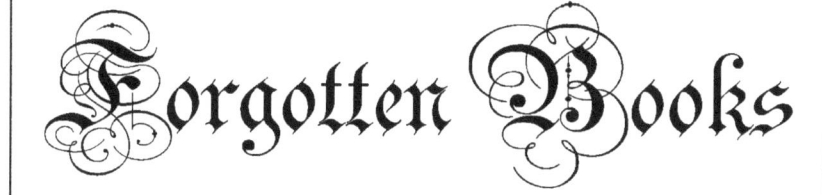

Forgotten Books

www.ForgottenBooks.com

Read online
Download PDF
Purchase in print

ISBN 978-1-330-38019-2
PIBN 10045680

This book is a reproduction of an important historical work. Forgotten Books uses state-of-the-art technology to digitally reconstruct the work, preserving the original format whilst repairing imperfections present in the aged copy. In rare cases, an imperfection in the original, such as a blemish or missing page, may be replicated in our edition. We do, however, repair the vast majority of imperfections successfully; any imperfections that remain are intentionally left to preserve the state of such historical works.

Forgotten Books is a registered trademark of FB &c Ltd.
Copyright © 2018 FB &c Ltd.
FB &c Ltd, Dalton House, 60 Windsor Avenue, London, SW19 2RR.
Company number 08720141. Registered in England and Wales.

For support please visit www.forgottenbooks.com

1 MONTH OF FREE READING

at
www.ForgottenBooks.com

By purchasing this book you are eligible for one month membership to ForgottenBooks.com, giving you unlimited access to our entire collection of over 1,000,000 titles via our web site and mobile apps.

To claim your free month visit: www.forgottenbooks.com/free45680

* Offer is valid for 45 days from date of purchase. Terms and conditions apply.

English
Français
Deutsche
Italiano
Español
Português

www.forgottenbooks.com

Mythology Photography **Fiction**
Fishing Christianity **Art** Cooking
Essays Buddhism Freemasonry
Medicine **Biology** Music **Ancient Egypt** Evolution Carpentry Physics
Dance Geology **Mathematics** Fitness
Shakespeare **Folklore** Yoga Marketing
Confidence Immortality Biographies
Poetry **Psychology** Witchcraft
Electronics Chemistry History **Law**
Accounting **Philosophy** Anthropology
Alchemy Drama Quantum Mechanics
Atheism Sexual Health **Ancient History**
Entrepreneurship Languages Sport
Paleontology Needlework Islam
Metaphysics Investment Archaeology
Parenting Statistics Criminology
Motivational

The Treatment of War Wounds

By

W. W. Keen, M.D., LL.D.

Major, Medical Reserve Corps, U. S. Army
Emeritus Professor of Surgery
Jefferson Medical College, Philadelphia

Second Edition, Reset

Philadelphia and London
W. B. SAUNDERS COMPANY
1918

Copyright, 1917, by W. B. Saunders Company. Reprinted December, 1917.
Revised, entirely reset, reprinted, and recopyrighted May, 1918

Copyright, 1918, by W. B. Saunders Company

PRINTED IN AMERICA

PREFATORY NOTE TO THE SECOND EDITION

The speedy exhaustion of the first edition of this little book has necessitated this second edition only about six months after the first was issued. The rapid progress made in the treatment of war wounds through clinical observation, but more especially by the active research work at the front, as well as at base hospitals and laboratories in England, France, and the United States, has been such that this edition is almost a new book, so largely has it been rewritten. The type has been entirely reset.

The large space now given to shock, to the Carrel-Dakin and other methods of treatment, to fractures, tetanus, wounds of the head, chest, and joints, to gas gangrene, the Bull-Pritchett serum, orthopedic surgery, etc., will be welcomed, I am sure. The introduction of résumés of some of the more important papers, with appended short bibliographies, which will enable the reader to obtain fuller information, will commend themselves to those who wish for more.

Even more fully than before I have had the efficient and welcome aid of experts in various special subjects, to whom my warm thanks are due. Among

10 PREFATORY NOTE TO THE SECOND EDITION

these I gladly name Dr. Alexis Carrel and his assistants, Lt. Glenn E. Cullen, Dr. G. Loewy, Dr. G. Dehelly, and Mrs. J. M. Doane, also Drs. W. T. Porter, H. D. Dakin, and Captains W. Estell Lee and W. H. Furness, and the writers of the personal letters at the end of the volume, especially to Sir Anthony A. Bowlby, Bart.; also to Miss Ida W. Pritchett, for aid in the section on gas infection and gas gangrene.

Dr. Dawson Williams, editor of the British Medical Journal, has also given me valued assistance. To his kindness I owe the large chart of the Thomas and other splints, one of the publications of the British medical officials, from which are reproduced Figs. 7–20. He also granted permission to use Figs. 47 to 52 from Major Harvey Cushing's article in the British Medical Journal, as I had not the opportunity to ask that of Major Cushing. For the chapter on the Localization and Removal of Foreign Bodies I am indebted, with the permission of Surgeon General W. C. Gorgas, to Major John S. Shearer, of the New York School of Military Roentgenology, and Dr. David R. Bowen, of the Jefferson Medical College. I am particularly glad that they included parts of the section on the same subject in the first edition, describing Major E. W. Caldwell's ingenious apparatus, soon to be tested

PREFATORY NOTE TO THE SECOND EDITION 11

To keep abreast of the rapidly improving means of treatment of war wounds, of course, the leading journals in the allied countries are indispensable.

Masson & Cie, Paris, have announced over thirty manuals under the general title "*Collection Horizon.*" Almost all have been already published; a number of them have been translated into English.

Major A. J. Hull, R.A.M.C., has published a valuable manual entitled "*Surgery in War.*"

Lea and Febiger, Philadelphia, have announced a series of "*Medical War Manuals,*" issued under the supervision of the Surgeon General and the Council of National Defense. Five of these have already appeared.

I cordially commend also Depage's L'Ambulance de l'Océan (Masson & Cie, Paris), and the "Medical Bulletin of the Red Cross" in France, 6 Rue Piccini, Paris. This was begun in November, 1917; is issued monthly, and is distributed without cost to the medical officers in the allied armies and to others engaged in war relief work who may find it useful. Each number has a review of some important topic and abstracts from the more important articles in the current journals.

WILLIAM W. KEEN.

PHILADELPHIA,
 May, 1918.

PREFATORY NOTE TO THE FIRST EDITION

This Report has been much delayed by circumstances beyond my control. Happily the delay has had its compensations, as I have been enabled to add important matter from the large experience of several able surgeons actually in the conflict. I have been enabled also to include the work on Acriflavine, Proflavine and Brilliant Green, Mercurophen, and the latest technic on the Paraffin Treatment of Burns, etc., which were not published until recently.

But more especially am I gratified to be able to add, as the Report is passing through the press, two most important contributions to our knowledge—one, the new antiseptic, Dichloramin-T, and the simplified technic of Dakin for the treamtent of infection in wounds; and the other the most welcome announcement of an antitoxin against gas gangrene. This will be indeed a boon to many.

I should have quoted Carrel and Dehelly (Le Traitement des Plaies infectees) and Dumas and Carrel (Pratique de l'Irrigation des Plaies dans la Methode du Docteur Carrel) directly, but unfortunately I was not able to obtain copies of these books until just after I had completed the text. I have, however, been able to utilize some cuts from Carrel and Dehelly by the kind permission of the authors and of Messrs. Masson & Cie, of Paris. I have reproduced some illustrations from the British Medical Journal of June 9, 1917, from a paper by Bowlby. The editor of the Journal gave his permission to use these, but I had to assume that of Sir Anthony, as it was impossible to wait for his permission. I have also to thank Colonel Thomas H. Goodwin, of the British Army, and the Editor of the Journal of the American Medical Association, for permission to use Fig. 4, the diagram from Colonel Goodwin's paper.

WILLIAM W. KEEN

CONTENTS

	PAGE
RESPECTS IN WHICH PRESENT WAR DIFFERS FROM PREVIOUS WARS	17
HUGE NUMBERS IN CONTENDING ARMIES	19
SHOCK	22
NEW MEANS OF TRANSPORTATION OF WOUNDED	37
FRACTURES	46
Bibliography on Orthopedics, 60.	
NEW WEAPONS	62
THE CARREL-DAKIN METHOD	86
Dakin's Hypochlorite Solution, 87; Preparation, 89; Preparation from Chlorin and Sodium Carbonate, 90; Preparation from Bleaching Powder and Sodium Carbonate, 91; Preparation of Daufresne Chloramin-T Paste, 93; Technic of Dressing—Necessary Materials, 95; Preparing Wound for Introduction of Antiseptic, 97; Introduction of Instillation Tubes, 99; Aftercare of Wounds, 102; Bacteriologic Examination of Wound, 103; Reunion of Wound, 104; Objections to Method, 109.	
DICHLORAMIN-T	111
Technic, 114.	
THE "BIPP" TREATMENT OF MR. RUTHERFORD MORISON	118
LOCALIZATION AND REMOVAL OF FOREIGN BODIES BY X-RAYS	123
Localization of Foreign Bodies, 123; Fluoroscopic Assistance During Operation, 137; Stereo-fluoroscopy, 140; Removal of Foreign Bodies, 144.	

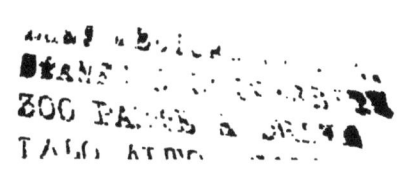

CONTENTS

                                                    PAGE

TETANUS.. 145
    Memorandum on Tetanus Issued by the British War Office Committee, 150; Specific Treatment, 156; Symptomatic Treatment, 160; Method of Performing Intrathecal Injection, 164.

GAS INFECTION AND GAS GANGRENE................... 166
    An Antitoxin to Prevent Gas Gangrene, 174.

HOSPITAL GANGRENE.. 177

WOUNDS OF THE HEAD...................................... 179

WOUNDS OF THE CHEST..................................... 199

WOUNDS OF THE JOINTS.................................... 210

ABDOMINAL WOUNDS.. 220

BURNS.. 231

PERSONAL LETTERS... 239
    Letter from Sir Anthony A. Bowlby, Bart., 240; Second Letter from Sir Anthony A. Bowlby, Bart., 244; Letter from Major Joseph A. Blake, 248; Letter from Major George W. Crile, 251; Letter from Dr. William S. Halsted, 252; Letter from Dr. Victor G. Heiser, 259.

BIBLIOGRAPHY ON REHABILITATION OF CRIPPLED SOLDIERS. FURNISHED BY MAJOR R. TAIT MCKENZIE, R.A.M.C. 260

APPENDIX... 262
    The "Cotton-Process" Ether, p. 262.
    Anesthesia During Dressing of Wounds, 264.

INDEX... 265

THE TREATMENT OF WAR WOUNDS

This Report has been compiled at the request of the National Research Council, and especially of its Medical Committee, of which Dr. Victor C. Vaughan is Chairman. It does not pretend to be complete, but is only a memorandum on some of the more important and most recent improvements in the treatment of war wounds.

Unfortunately, my knowledge is necessarily second-hand, as I have been unable to visit the hospitals in Europe; but letters from a number of my friends who have had first-hand experience, which I solicited and print herewith, are most valuable documents, covering a number of subjects of importance: some of them medical, besides war wounds proper. My hearty thanks are tendered to them, especially to those who have taken time in their overworked lives to furnish this valuable information. Theirs is indeed first-hand knowledge. In a few pregnant sentences they express convictions which are the result of hard and sometimes bitter experiences of months and even years of warfare. Even in those letters differences of opinion are seen.

From the surgical point of view, the present war differs widely from any preceding wars in five principal respects:

(1) The huge numbers in the armies and, therefore, of the wounded.

(2) The new means of transportation.

(3) The new weapons, especially in the artillery.

(4) Rampant infection of wounds.

(5) The conquest of infection by more efficient antiseptics and by new methods.

In three additional respects also great progress has been made:

(a) The reconstructive surgery of the face and jaws by the coöperation of the dentist and the surgeon, (b) the great development of war orthopedics, and (c) the training of disabled soldiers. These topics I must omit.

I should also call attention to one strange means of preventing wounds, which, though neither surgical nor medical, yet is of great practical value.

We are apparently returning to the use of steel armor, as in the middle ages. Light steel helmets and to some extent corselets over the chest have undoubtedly lessened to a very appreciable extent wounds of the head and the thoracic viscera. In trench warfare the head is especially exposed, and here the helmet has found its chief use. Surgeons at the front testify to a marked diminution in the number of wounds of the head since the introduction of steel helmets.

The **huge numbers** in the contending armies cause sudden flooding of the hospitals, especially those near the front, with enormous numbers of the wounded after each "drive" or assault. Thus a hospital with 300 or 400 beds may suddenly be overwhelmed by 1000 or more cases.

One of the objections urged against the Carrel-Dakin method is that when such numbers overwhelm the staff, it is impossible to take the time necessary for the exact technic which this method requires. Whether this objection is valid in such emergencies I cannot judge, for I have had no personal experience. From what I have learned, both by reading and by the personal account given to me by those who *have* had experience, were I in France I should institute this method and adhere to it until compelled to abandon it and substitute other more speedy methods. Depage, with a hospital of 800 beds, very near the firing line and, therefore, especially liable to such sudden floods of patients, from what I can learn, seems to be able to use the method efficiently. (*Cf.* pp. 81–83.)

It is often physically impossible to give speedy and thorough treatment to *all* patients. A single case, even if it urgently requires attention,—if this will absorb a long time,—may have to wait, for in that same time a dozen others, almost equally exigent, but requiring less time, might be cared for. The greatest good of the greatest number must be the rule. On the other hand, an abdominal case or a case of internal hemorrhage, even if it does involve time, must have precedence of a dozen who can wait. The surgeon's good judgment must be his constant guide.

Walters and three colleagues,* as a result of 500 emergency operations, make an excellent suggestion, which I believe has been already carried into effect, viz., the establishment of an "observation ward" for "doubtful" cases. If they are mixed with others, they may easily be overlooked in the rush of wounded during and immediately after an active engagement. In this ward each case should be tagged with his surgeon's name, and at frequent intervals each surgeon should visit his own doubtful cases and be ready to seize the favorable moment should it come.

* Lancet, February 10, 1917.

"Take invariably men in the best condition and most hopeful *first*," and leave other cases for further consideration, is their prudent advice, or, as Webb and Milligan, in an excellent paper full of good sense,[*] put it, to spend time on moribund cases is time wasted: on those not moribund, is time well used.

For the same reason, and for want of the needed aseptic conditions, few abdominal cases and few if any injuries involving the brain were operated on near the front during the early period of the war.

Shock from severe wounds and hemorrhage, however, always must take precedence of everything else.

As the war has progressed, especially on the western front, where the trench lines have been relatively fixed for months, the stations and hospitals near the front have gradually become far better equipped and abdominal and severe cerebral cases have been more frequently operated on.

[*] Brit. Jour. Surg., iv.

SHOCK

W. T. Porter,* in a graphic and illuminating report on "Shock at the Front," from observations made as perilously near as within 38 meters of the German trenches, and during a second longer visit (see his delightful book, "Shock at the Front," Atlantic Monthly Press, Boston, 1918), has especially called attention to shock and to the great saving of life which would result if the same means which have been proved effective in experimental research in animals were adopted in man.

He has kindly furnished me with a summary which I reproduce in part as follows:

"The critical level of blood-pressure is that point below which the blood-pressure will not usually rise again without assistance. The critical level of the diastolic pressure was close to 60 mm., on the scale of the Vaquez sphygmomanometer used by me in France.

"An understanding of the critical level is of the first importance in the study and treatment of shock.

* Boston Med. and Surg. Jour., December 14, 1916.

If the blood-pressure just touches the critical level, a difference of ten millimeters of mercury may be the difference between life and death. A few millimeters above this level, recovery will usually occur spontaneously; a few millimeters below, death will follow unless skilled aid be at hand. . . .

"In the summer of 1916, during my service in the fighting line in France, I learned that in this war shock occurs chiefly after shell fractures of the femur and after multiple wounds through the subcutaneous fat. In 1000 casualties observed by me at the Massif de Moronvillers, these were the only injuries producing shock, except certain abdominal wounds in which the shell fragments undoubtedly disturbed the vasomotor apparatus of the largest vascular area in the body.

"It has long been known that fat embolism takes place after fractures of the thigh and after multiple wounds through the subcutaneous fat.

"In February, 1917, I proved that the injection of a small quantity of neutral olive oil in the jugular vein was followed by a falling blood-pressure and the other symptoms of traumatic shock. The resulting publication (Boston Med. and Surg. Jour., 1917, clxxvi, p. 248) was the first clear statement that shock as seen on the battle-field is usually caused by fat embolism.

"Shortly thereafter I developed a new remedy for the treatment of shock. All physiologists know that the pumping action of the diaphragm is an important aid in the movement of blood from the abdomen into the chest. At the height of a strong inspiration the venous pressure in the chest may be more than 40 millimeters lower than the venous pressure in the abdomen. I produced strong respiratory movements of the diaphragm by allowing the animal to breathe an atmosphere rich in carbon dioxid. The *diastolic* arterial pressure [which should always be the guide: the systolic pressure should not be used as the standard] was thereby increased 15 and even 30 millimeters. (*Ibid.*, p. 699.)

"In June, 1917, I successfully applied this new method to the treatment of wounded soldiers.* In cases almost pulseless, cases in which all other means of raising the blood-pressure had failed, the carbon dioxid respiration strengthened the pulse and raised the diastolic blood-pressure 10 millimeters. This rise is of great value when the pressure is at the critical level.

"The general treatment employed by me at the Chemin des Dames was as follows: A shock room was made next the operating room. The patient was

* *Ibid.*, 1917, clxxvii, p. 326.

carried to the shock room directly from the ambulance. He was not washed. He was at once placed on an operating table, inclined so that the feet were 30 cm. higher than the head. An electric heater was put between the blankets and the body. The diastolic pressure was taken every fifteen minutes. Where indicated, injections of warm normal saline solution were made into a vein and carbon dioxid respiration was employed. If his state was grave, adrenalin was added to the saline solution. When his condition justified operation, the clothing was cut away about the wound and the area disinfected; neighboring regions were covered with sterile cloths. He was then moved, still in the inclined position, and still on his hot table, to the operating room. The operation was done under local anesthesia whenever possible. At its close the patient was wheeled back to the shock room, still on the same inclined hot table. I did not leave him until he was out of danger or dead. Repeated readings of the pressure were taken. The remedies were directed to raising the diastolic pressure to a point about 15 millimeters above the critical level—more is not necessary. Carbon dioxid respiration was frequently employed, and always with benefit. One case was operated on during the carbon dioxid breathing, with apparent advantage.

"Under these methods four-fifths of the patients recovered."

[Whatever may be thought of the theoretical basis for Porter's treatment of shock, a treatment which gives a recovery rate of 80 per cent. surely deserves a thorough trial.—K.]

"A word as to details may be of interest. Normal saline solution should be injected at 39° C. (102.2° F.) measured by a thermometer in the vertical limb of a ⊥ tube placed next the cannula. If the pressure has not remained too long below the critical level, it will be raised by the normal saline; otherwise not, because the permeability of the vessel walls is increased by prolonged low pressure. Professor Bayliss states that the addition of 5 per cent. of gum arabic to the saline solution will prevent leakage and thus raise the pressure under all circumstances. This suggestion was made after my leaving France, and I have had no personal experience of its value. [The British Shock Investigating Committee recommends 6 per cent. of gum and 2 per cent. of sodium bicarbonate in place of sodium chlorid.—K.]

"Adrenalin is of temporary advantage, but even this fleeting rise of blood-pressure may save life. In the laboratory the blood-pressure of animals may be raised for considerable periods by allowing the well-diluted adrenalin to flow into the vein drop by drop from a buret. I have not tried this on men.

"Dr. Meltzer very recently stated that the pressor action of epinephrin is much prolonged when the drug is injected into the vertebral canal.

"To give the carbon dioxid, the head of the patient was placed in a wooden box, 25 cm. broad, 30 cm. high, and 30 cm. long. The end for the neck was in two pieces. The lower piece was fixed and had a semicircular opening for the back of the neck. The upper piece was movable. It had a semicircular opening for the front of the neck. This piece slid down upon the neck like a guillotine. Cotton was placed between the edges of the openings and the skin. A hole of about 2 cm. in diameter was made in each of the two sides of the box. Cotton was placed in these holes to regulate the amount of carbon dioxid and air. The carbon dioxid entered one of these holes. It came from a cylinder provided with a regulating valve. On its way it bubbled through a water bottle. The volume of gas employed was judged by the number of bubbles per minute. Enough gas was used to double the respiration.

"The carbon dioxid respiration should not be stopped too abruptly.

"If acidosis be suspected, I am told by eminent

authority that 5 grams of sodium bicarbonate should be injected into a vein and the urine be drawn from the bladder. After an hour the reaction of the freshly secreted urine should be taken. If it is alkaline, acidosis may be excluded, for the time at least. If acid, the urine should again be drawn, and 10 grams of sodium bicarbonate be injected into a vein. If after an hour the newly excreted urine is still acid, more sodium bicarbonate can be given by the mouth. I have not studied this treatment personally."

In the Journal of the American Medical Association for February 23 and March 2, 1918, are six extremely important and elaborate articles by Cowell, Hooper, Fraser, and Cannon, members of the Special Committee of the British General Research Committee to Investigate Shock.

The Committee consists of ten distinguished men, of whom two, Cannon, of Boston, and A. N. Richards, of Philadelphia, are Americans. These articles have been reprinted as a pamphlet to be had of the Journal for ten cents. No résumé or satisfactory abstract can be made. As this book is concerned especially with treatment, I am compelled to omit theories of the causation of shock unless capable of brief statement (*e. g.*, Porter's).

The last paper of the six is by Cannon, and is a

practical paper on the "Preventive Treatment of Wound Shock." Its importance is such that every surgeon should read it carefully. I can give only the most important details. Whatever is the nature of wound shock "it is evident that the circulatory functions are in a precarious condition, and that the heart, nervous system, and other organs are suffering from an insufficient blood supply." The other papers in the series show that—

1. Cooling of the body lowers still further an already low blood-pressure or keeps it at a low level.

2. Operation on a patient in shock "is accompanied by a rapid and large increase of an acidosis which is already present, and by a correspondingly sudden and extensive fall in an existent low arterial pressure."

A patient wounded in the *front line trenches* may reach aid quickly, but on the contrary he may easily be one to two hours away from the first-aid station. Of course, the very first thing to be done even before he is carried away is to arrest hemorrhage often by a tourniquet and apply first-aid dressings to prevent sepsis. A well-trained orderly may administer ¼ grain of morphin by the mouth,* and then carry him as gently as possible to the first-aid station.

* [Morphin should be given by preference hypodermically for evident reasons, but it may easily be impossible to do so.—K.]

"To send blankets to all parts of the line is impossible, but by the adoption of a waterproof sheet-blanket 'packet' system a stretcher prepared for use is provided with means for preventing excessive loss of body heat. Reference to Fig. 1 will make clear this simple method of carrying a dry blanket. This method has already been put into practice in a large part of the line.

"All regimental stretchers at advanced bearer posts in the front line, and stretchers carried by working parties, should be equipped with this packet. The regimental bearers should be insistently instructed by their medical officer as to the importance of doing everything to prevent wound shock. The wounded man should be guarded as much as possible against loss of heat. Efficient first-aid should be given rapidly without unduly exposing the patient to the cold for a prolonged period. A hot drink should be given at the earliest moment. Then, having been carefully wrapped up, the patient should be carried down with all speed to the regimental aid post. . . .

"At the *regimental aid post* it is wise to consider the general condition of the patient first and his wound second. A dry stretcher with three blankets should always be in readiness for a possible case at any time of the day or night. . . .

"Space will be limited; but an open stretcher, together with three blankets folded lengthwise three times, may be kept supported horizontally against the wall of the dugout behind the stove (Fig. 2).

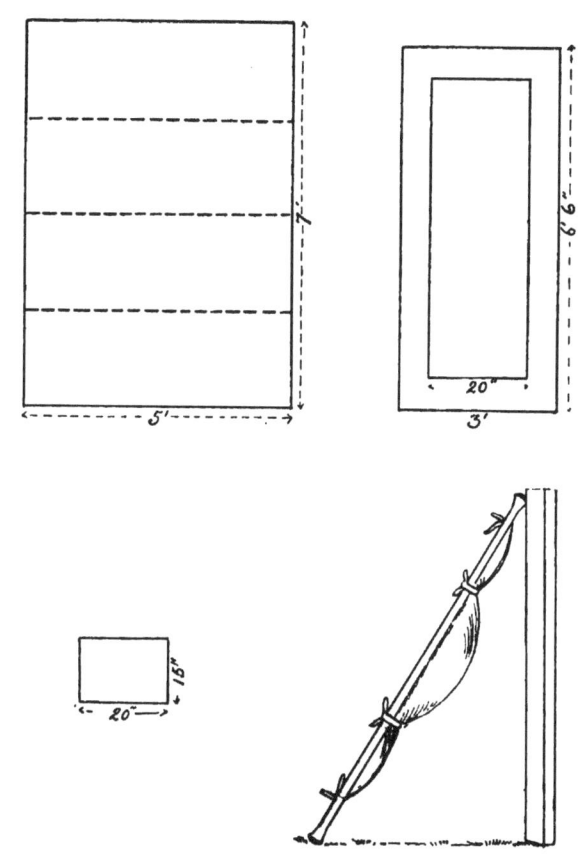

Fig. 1.—Method of carrying a dry blanket (Cannon, Fraser, and Cowell).

A dry stretcher and a supply of warm blankets will thus always be at hand. A tin of water may be kept standing on the fire to provide for hot drinks and for filling hot-water bottles.

"As soon as a patient arrives he should be given a few ounces of hot drink, and his wet boots and puttees removed, along with any other clothing which may cover wounds. Meanwhile the dry stretcher is prepared by arranging the first two blankets so that four folds will come underneath the patient (Fig. 2). The blankets are covered temporarily

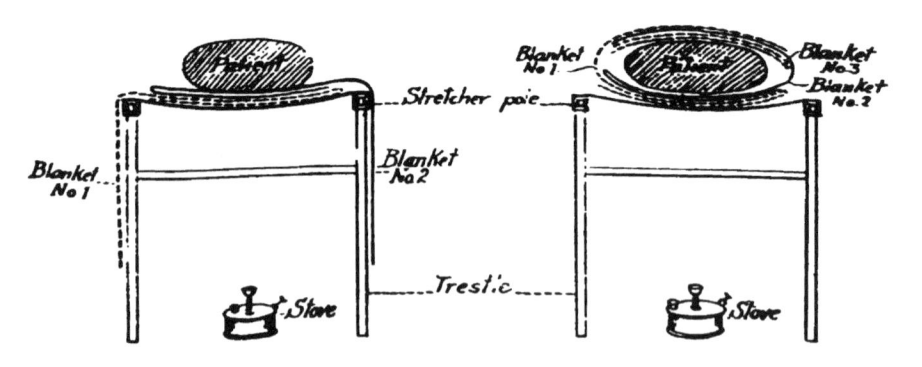

Fig. 2.—Method of folding three blankets to give four folds above and below the patient; also the formation of a hot-air chamber (Cannon, Fraser, and Cowell).

with a waterproof sheet to prevent soiling while wounds are being dressed. The man is now transferred to this prepared stretcher, which is supported on trestles and stands well over the stove. The third or free fold of each of the lower two blankets hangs down on either side and helps to form an enclosed warming chamber. If there is no constant source of heat, a hot-air chamber may be made in a few minutes by use of a Primus or Beatrice stove.*

"The patient is now becoming warmed, while the medical officer is attending to the surgical cleansing of the wounds and neighboring parts, and is applying proper dressings and splints. As soon as the dressings are finished, well-guarded hot-water bottles are placed in each axilla and a third across the loins or between the legs; and the third blanket, which is doubled lengthwise, is laid over the patient. The two warmed blankets which have been hanging to form the sides of the hot-air chamber are lifted, carried over the patient, and tucked in. He now has four folds of blanket over him as well as underneath.

"Finally, just before the patient is sent off, he is given a hot drink of sweetened tea in which a dram of sodium bicarbonate is dissolved."

At the *advanced dressing station* any necessary treatment [*e. g.*, including an antitetanic injection.—K.] and another alkaline drink are given, and hot-water bottles may be changed. He is then usually transported by motor or narrow gage railway to the field hospital, where heat is still applied as the most important part of the treatment of all serious cases.

* A Primus stove of ordnance pattern will burn a gallon of paraffin in twenty-four hours if operating continuously.

Here the patient is definitely operated on and may remain for some days or even longer.

It is easy to see that during a serious drive these details are carried out with difficulty. The best possible is aimed at, especially the ordinary surgical care mentioned and the *application of heat* and the *alkaline drinks.*

These are especially necessary if an operation has to be done. "Since acidosis develops in shock, . . . the recommendation is offered that wounded men be provided with a warm drink containing a dram or 4 grams of sodium bicarbonate at suitable relay posts on their way from the front to casualty clearing stations."

Instead of injecting warm saline, which may even increase the danger of acidosis, Cannon proposes an intravenous injection of a 4 per cent. solution of sodium bicarbonate, which is hypertonic. It should, therefore, be introduced slowly, say one ounce a minute. It should be delivered into the vein at a few degrees above normal body temperature. If a tube of considerable length is used, the temperature should be from 110° to 115° F. *The solution must not be boiled,* as that changes the bicarbonate to the carbonate. Both the water and the salt employed, as well as the instruments, hands, etc., should be sterile. The injection should be begun at the start of the anesthetic.

"An alkaline injection at the start of anesthesia prevents the dangerous depressive effects which the anesthetic and operative procedures have in cases of shock with acidosis. The operation ends, not with an increase of the existent acidosis, but with the acidosis overcome and a normal alkaline reserve provided. And the blood-pressure, instead of being perilously lowered, is actually raised during the critical period."

Much of this treatment is already in effect.

The chief drawback, it seems to me, is the amount of time which must be given to the individual patient. During a great "drive" it may be difficult or even impossible to give so much time to one man.

On the other hand, Porter states that such shock cases number only about one in 100. When possible, the results prove it to be time well spent, for "men who looked like cadavers and were almost pulseless came back to life and after two hours talked pleasantly of their children."

Bowlby calls attention to the fact that the wounded will often have suffered from loss of blood, loss of sleep, insufficient food, and exposure to cold, and if to these are added severe pain and the exhaustion due to an unavoidable jolting transportation, they will be on the verge of collapse. The first needs of such a man are *rest, warmth,* and *food,* of which the first two are the most important. These restoratives may easily be required before any treatment (save for hemorrhage) should be attempted. "The more experienced the surgeon, the less is he likely to hurry on a severe primary amputation." Threatened gas gangrene or rapidly spreading sepsis may force his hand. Much discretion, therefore, must be allowed the surgeon.

Archibald and Maclean* emphasize the need for warmth by stating that in their cases of profound shock the ordinary clinical thermometer did not register low enough, as in some of their the temperature was below 92° F. G. Holmes, in injuries of the cord at the sixth to the eighth cervical segments, has observed temperatures of 80° F., yet the patients survived for several days.

* Trans. Amer. Surg. Assoc., 1917.

TRANSPORTATION

The new means of transportation by automobile has helped enormously. While the wounded must often lie for hours and sometimes days in the "No Man's Land" between the opposing trenches, and the removal of the wounded must be done largely at night, yet, on the whole, they have been brought to hospitals, as at La Panne to Depage, and at Compiègne to Carrel, often within a few hours—sometimes within less than an hour.

There is an exhaustive technical paper on the Automobile Ambulance Service in the *Military Surgeon* for October, 1917. It is based on nineteen months' experience with the French army. To show how efficient this service was he states (p. 426) that during two months, in a division numbering 28,000 men, "no case was kept waiting" and he knew of "several cases which were actually on the operating table in a hospital in between thirty-five and forty minutes after being wounded." This whole paper will well repay very careful study by all connected with the Ambulance Service.

Later, attention will be called to the rapidity with which infection spreads, and therefore the overwhelming importance of the earliest possible removal of the wounded to hospitals, where tetanus, gas infection, and other infections can be prevented, ameliorated, or cured. Hence the means of quick transportation are so important that I have included this as seriously contributing to the proper wound treatment.

The diagram on page 39, kindly furnished me by Colonel Henry Page, of the United States Army Medical Corps, shows at a glance the scheme of the American army, the different zones of collection, evacuation, distribution; the various kinds of hospitals; the personnel which serves these hospitals, and the means of transportation in each zone. This will save a long description. Compare the diagrams on pages 39 and 40.

It should be noted, as pointed out by Colonel Page, that this plan of charging the Medical Department with the orderly transportation of the wounded from the front, where they were a burden to the fighting forces and where surgical treatment was impossible, to where such treatment was possible, is due to the foresight and administrative ability of Jonathan Letterman, my old Chief and Medical Director of the Army of the Potomac in 1862. He was one of

TRANSPORTATION

the remarkable military medical men developed by the Civil War.

ZONES OF COLLECTION, EVACUATION, AND DISTRIBUTION IN THE UNITED STATES ARMY

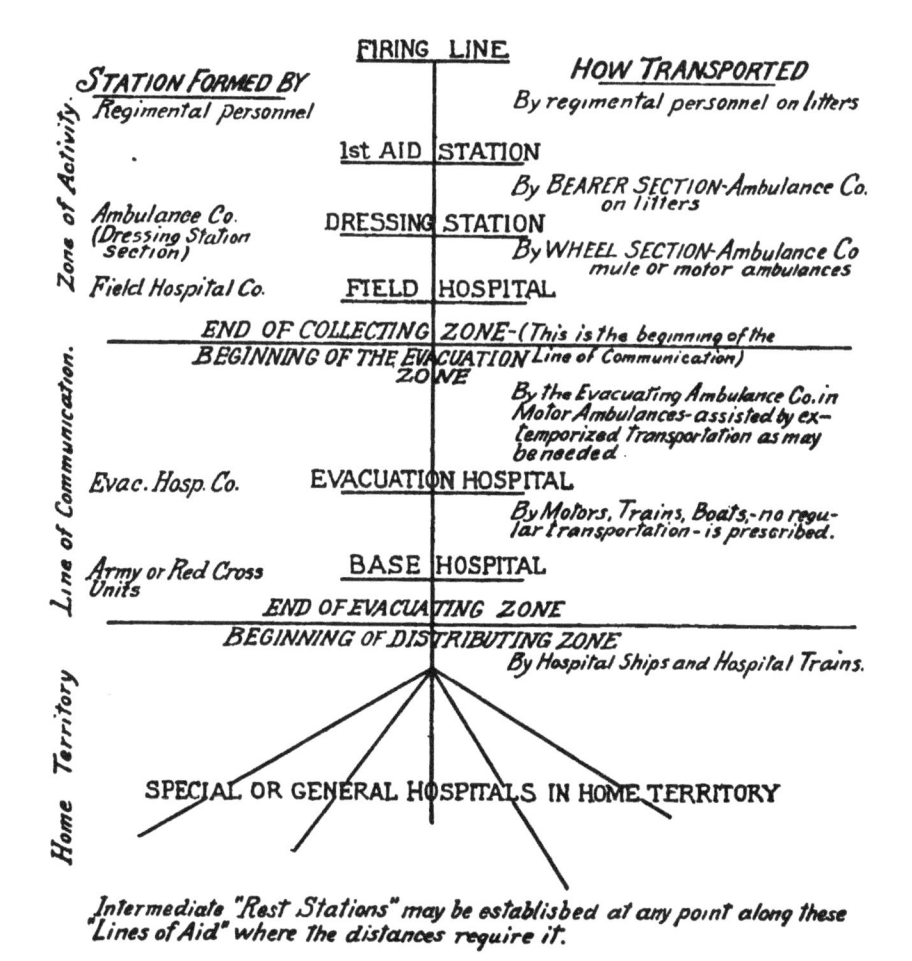

```
                              FIRING LINE
     STATION FORMED BY                     HOW TRANSPORTED
       Regimental personnel              By regimental personnel on litters
                              1st AID STATION
                                         By BEARER SECTION-Ambulance Co.
       Ambulance Co.                              on litters
       (Dressing Station     DRESSING STATION
        Section)                         By WHEEL SECTION-Ambulance Co
       Field Hospital Co.                      mule or motor ambulances
                              FIELD HOSPITAL
           END OF COLLECTING ZONE-(This is the beginning of the
           BEGINNING OF THE EVACUATION Line of Communication)
                                  ZONE
                                         By the Evacuating Ambulance Co. in
                                         Motor Ambulances-assisted by ex-
                                         temporized transportation as may
                                         be needed
       Evac. Hosp. Co.        EVACUATION HOSPITAL
                                         By Motors, Trains, Boats,-no regu-
                                         lar transportation-is prescribed.
       Army or Red Cross      BASE HOSPITAL
       Units
                        END OF EVACUATING ZONE
                        BEGINNING OF DISTRIBUTING ZONE
                                         By Hospital Ships and Hospital Trains.


            SPECIAL OR GENERAL HOSPITALS IN HOME TERRITORY
```

Intermediate "Rest Stations" may be established at any point along these "Lines of Aid" where the distances require it.

Fig. 3.—Colonel Page's diagram (U. S. Army).

By the kind permission of Colonel Thomas H. Goodwin, C.M.G., D.S.O., now (April, 1918) Director General of the Medical Service of the British Army, and of the editor of the Journal of the American

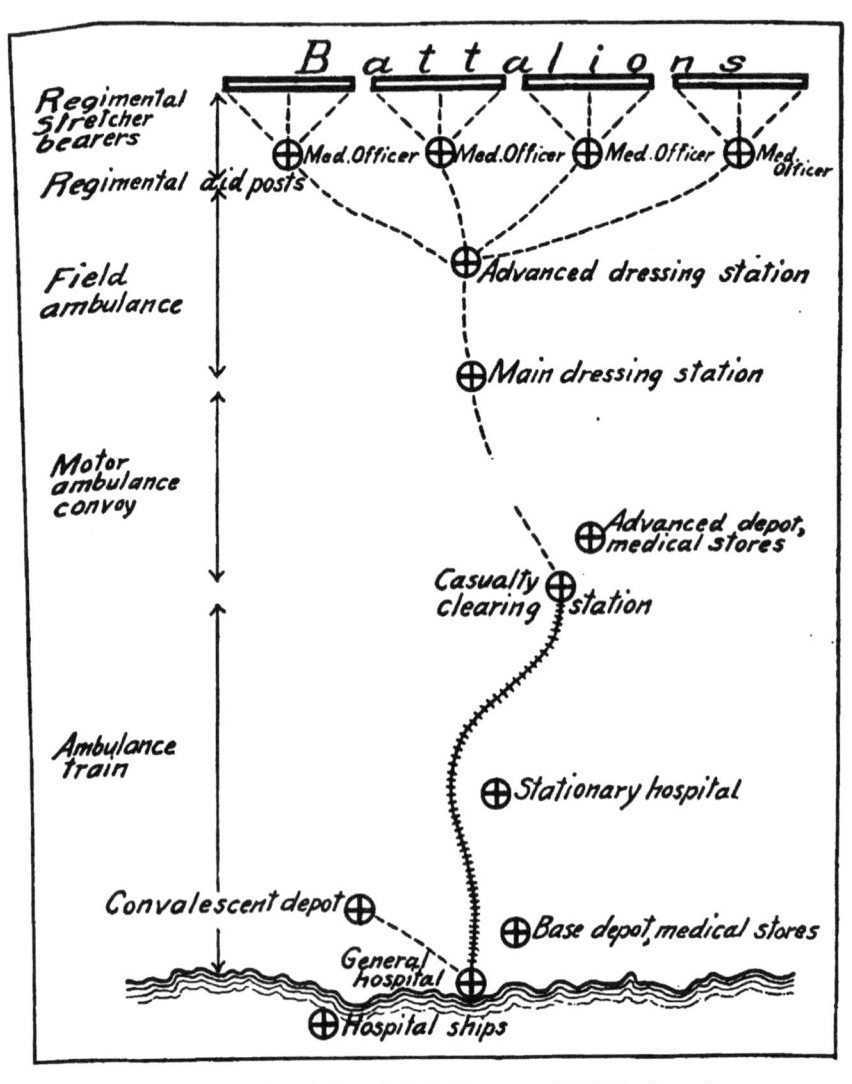

Fig. 4.—Colonel Goodwin's diagram (British Army).

Medical Association (July 14, 1917), I am enabled to add a corresponding diagram showing the relation of similar hospitals in the British Army. The average distances, Colonel Goodwin states, are as follows: The "Regimental Medical Officer" will be about 500 yards behind the front trenches; further back, in succession, (1) to the "advanced dressing stations" will be half a mile to a mile, (2) to the "main dressing station" a mile and a half more, and (3) to the "casualty clearing station" (C. C. S.), say, five miles further.

At the first-aid station, and possibly at the dressing station, only urgent operations should be done, especially, *e. g.*, for the arrest of hemorrhage. No patient should ever be forwarded from the C. C. S. with a tourniquet still applied on a limb. In his admirable paper on "British Surgery at the Front"* Bowlby advises the amputation of "completely smashed limbs," and the retention of such patients, for at least a day, at what I presume will correspond to our dressing station or our field hospital. Whether this is practicable must be decided by the responsible surgeon in each case, for local, personal, and military conditions vary too much for a hard and fast rule.

His recommendation that abdominal cases and those severe cases requiring such care as cannot be given at this first-aid station should be forwarded to

* Brit. Med. Jour., June 2, 1917, p. 705.

the dressing station ("casualty clearing station" of the British) at once by special motor ambulances, and not be kept waiting for the regular motor convoys leaving at scheduled time, is sound both from the surgical and the humanitarian standpoint. Moreover, as Bowlby points out, had sufficient of these motor ambulances been in use in the early months of the war, they would have saved very many of the wounded from being taken prisoners by the Germans. "The Motor Ambulance," as he forcibly and rightly puts it, "is the very foundation on which all our surgery at the front is based."

This whole article is full of most important matter and should not only be read, but be studied, by every military surgeon. I find it, on the whole, the best summary of the surgical treatment developed by the war up to May, 1917, which I have read. His later letter (p. 224) is also full of good practical information.

The *automobile* is indispensable. The American Field Ambulance in France alone, about a year ago, had 400 motor ambulances in service, and had transported 300,000 wounded. Probably now the number is far larger.

By turning the exhaust gases of the engine into a sheet-iron box placed in the floor of the body, "automobiles can be well heated. The heat can be turned on and off at will."*

This is now the rule in the British Ambulances. It may be also in the French and the American, but I am not informed as to them.

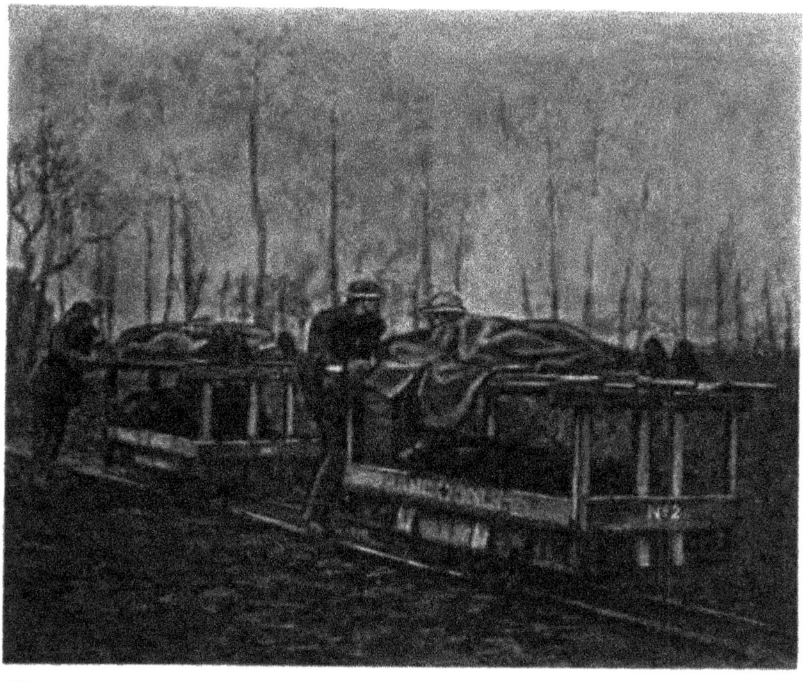

Fig. 5.—Light railway ambulance trolley (redrawn). (Kindness of the editor of the British Medical Journal and of Sir A. A. Bowlby, Bart. See Prefatory Note.)

Dr. Richard Cabot has called especial attention to the value of interchangeable standardized stretchers. In France an ambulance leaves the patients at the

* Thorn, *loc. cit.*, p. 419. See illustration in the Brit. Med. Jour., August 18, 1917, p. 224.

hospital lying on the stretchers, and receives exactly similar empty stretchers with their regular complement of blankets in exchange. This saves time and avoids transferring the patients to hospital stretchers, a process which often causes severe pain and adds to existing shock.

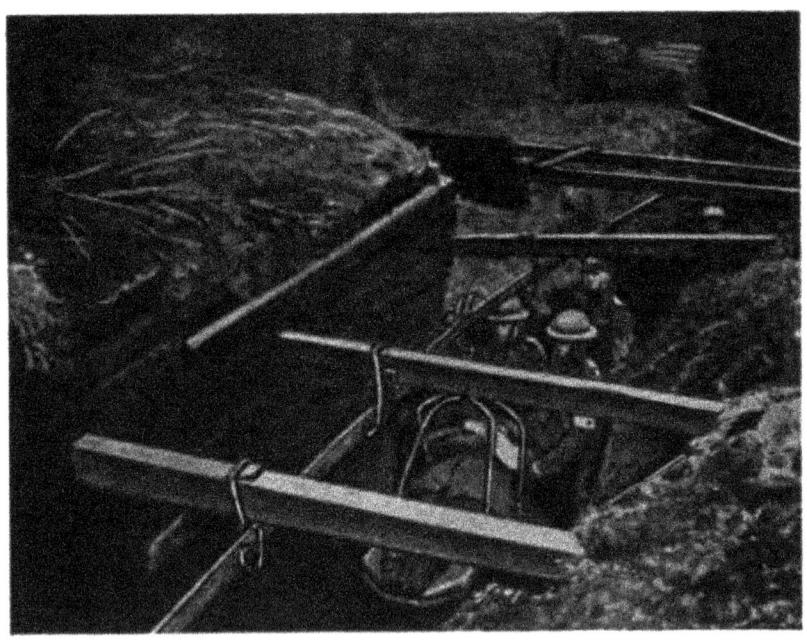

Fig. 6.—Overhead railway ambulance trolley (redrawn). (Kindness of the editor of the British Medical Journal and of Sir A. A. Bowlby, Bart.)

In what may be called the permanent trench warfare in France a light railway ambulance trolley (Fig. 5),* and even an overhead railway ambulance trolley (Fig. 6)* in the trenches for the rapid transportation of the wounded have been developed. These,

*Brit. Med. Jour., June 2, 1917, p. 711.

especially the overhead trolley, must be a great boon on account of the much smoother transportation.

The highly organized *hospital trains* in France, many of which are now in operation between the evacuation hospitals or C. C. S. and the base hospitals, are provided with permanent staffs of surgeons and nurses, with traveling laboratories, x-ray rooms, kitchens, and well-equipped operating-rooms. In France hospital barges on the canals, by their smoothness of transit, have been a blessing. Well-equipped hospital ships, especially across the Channel, have taken many thousands to permanent base hospitals in Great Britain, where the facilities are equal to the best.

Moynihan, during his recent American visit, laid especial emphasis on *immobility* in his usual trenchant style. He says (Jour. Amer. Med. Assoc., November 3, 1917, p. 1539): "The two things that have come out from all this exhaustive inquiry and most painstaking care of patients is that the primary essential is freedom of exposure of all parts [of the wound] through cleansing *and from first to last the most absolute immobility* that you can impose on any wound of the parts. It is just as important, or more important, to immobilize as firmly and as rigidly as you can a wound of the soft parts of the body, as a compound fracture of the bone."

FRACTURES

I can only briefly allude to *Fractures* because they demand full and detailed consideration for each fracture to be of much use, and that would be beyond the scope of this book.

I must, however, give space for a résumé of one very important address by Col. Sir Robert Jones,[*] together with a short bibliography of some of the more important orthopedic books and papers on the same topic, and a set of British drawings of the Thomas and some other splints (Figs. 7 to 20).

In this address on "The Orthopædic Outlook in Military Surgery," Sir Robert Jones gives what I think is the best résumé of the objects of the orthopedic surgeon and the qualities of what he calls the "orthopedic mind" that I have seen anywhere. "The orthopedic mind thinks in terms of function"— an admirable surgical aphorism. The address contains a number of very valuable suggestions as to orthopedic methods as they have developed during the war. He properly distinguishes between *pre-*

[*] Brit. Med. Jour., January 12, 1918.

ventive orthopedics and *corrective* orthopedics. The latter is more especially in the province of the orthopedic surgeon. *The former, however, lies in the province of almost every surgeon treating war wounds.* He especially emphasizes, in the department of preventive orthopedics, what he justly calls "the tragedy of the war"; namely, gunshot fractures of the femur.

The experience of the European army surgeons, and especially of such men as Sir Robert Jones and others in England, where they see the late results, have led them to urge that special hospitals, for example, for these fractures of the femur, should be established at accessible points and all cases of this injury be transferred as quickly as possible to such hospitals. The reason for this is very evident. Surgeons of special skill would be placed in charge of these hospitals, and their constantly accumulating experience would give them an immense advantage. Moreover, to such special hospitals younger and less skilled surgeons could be sent for special training by intensive short courses of instruction. Besides this, our brave soldiers are entitled to the very best skill and highest ability the nation can furnish.

This is what Surgeon General Hammond did at the suggestion of Weir Mitchell, during our Civil

War, on a small scale, but without the educational features just mentioned. There were special hospitals for wounds and diseases of the nervous system, for diseases and injuries of the eye, for diseases of the heart, etc.

Surgeon General Gorgas is planning such hospitals on a much larger scale.* It is proposed to have such hospitals as above described, and also for the ear, nose, and throat, for the mouth, face, and jaws, in which the dentists and the surgeons will coöperate, for orthopedic cases, for the repair, restoration, and reëducation of the disabled soldiers, who can thus be enabled to become in part or even wholly self-supporting.

Some of these special hospitals, *e. g.*, for injuries of the head, eye, fractures of the thigh, etc., must find their chief usefulness in or near the actual zone of fighting; others, as those for orthopedic repair and reëducation of the soldier, must be at the base or even in the United States. Still others will have to be established both in proximity to the fighting and also at the distant bases, so as to render immediate aid to those just wounded, and also to the convalescents far from the fighting zone.

* Jour. Amer. Med. Assoc., September 15, 1917.

The two fundamental principles of treating fractures of the femur, Sir Robert Jones says, are:

1. Efficient fixation in correct alinement at the earliest possible moment.

2. Continuity of treatment, *i. e.*, by the same surgeon, or at least at the same hospital.

To attain the first result he says that "there is no splint to compare with the Thomas'"

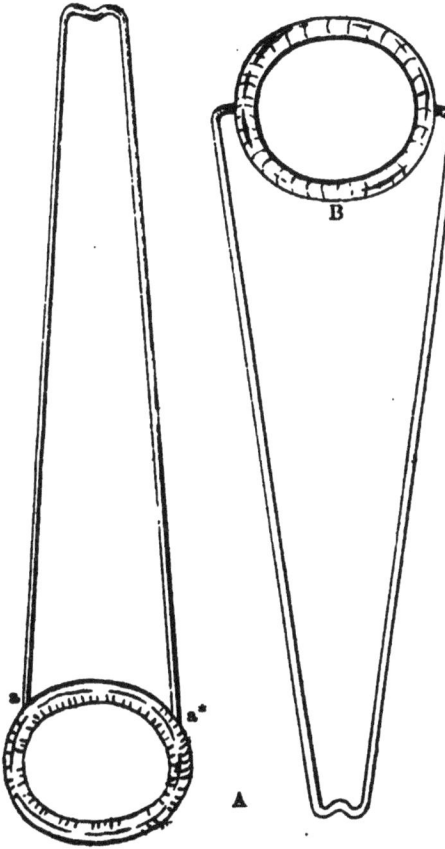

Fig. 7.—A, Thomas' splint for arm. This is bent to nearly a right angle at a a* for transport on a stretcher. B, Thomas' arm splint with swivel.

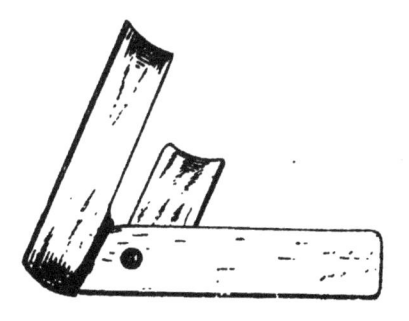

Fig. 8.—Bowlby's or Clarke's arm splint.

splint. With his enormous and successful experience this dictum should be accepted by everybody.

Osgood, of Boston,* describes in detail and with a number of cuts the modifications enabling one to use the "ring and wire" splints of Thomas and Sir Robert Jones, especially to the arm. "As surgeons become familiar with their use and appreciate the soundness of their simple mechanical principles, they are becoming more and more the method of choice, and the results obtained are becoming more perfect.

"The principle of extension by traction and counter-pressure makes of these splints a unit apparatus which provides easy and comfortable transportation, and allows the detailed treatment in the base and home hospitals to be continued with complete satisfaction without change of the apparatus, which may be, and now usually is, applied at the casualty clearing station or even at

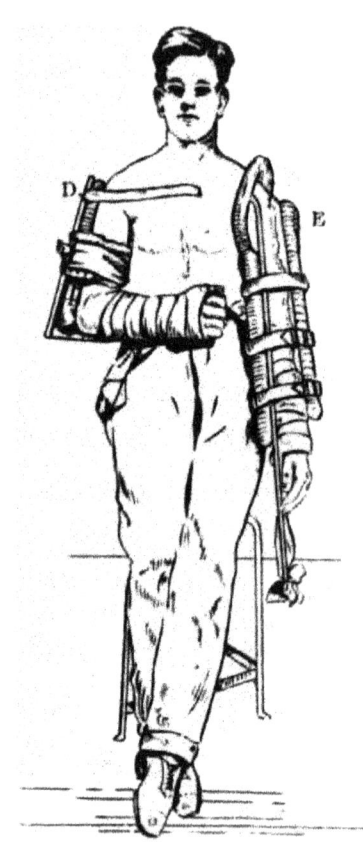

Fig. 9.—D, Bowlby's splint applied for fracture of right humerus. A narrow sling should also be used. E, Thomas' arm splint (bent near ring), applied for low fracture of left humerus.

* Brit. Med. Jour., October 13, 1917, p. 477.

Fig. 10.—Method of using Thomas' arm splint for fracture of leg bones in C. C. S. or base hospital only. The lower and upper strips of plaster make extension and counter-extension respectively, and are prevented from slipping by encircling bandage or plaster strapping. Perforated zinc or calico bandage slings support the fragments and popliteal space. Rotation of the foot is prevented by padding on each side or by a wire "foot piece." The splint is slung from a, a*, and b (Captain R. D. Laurie).

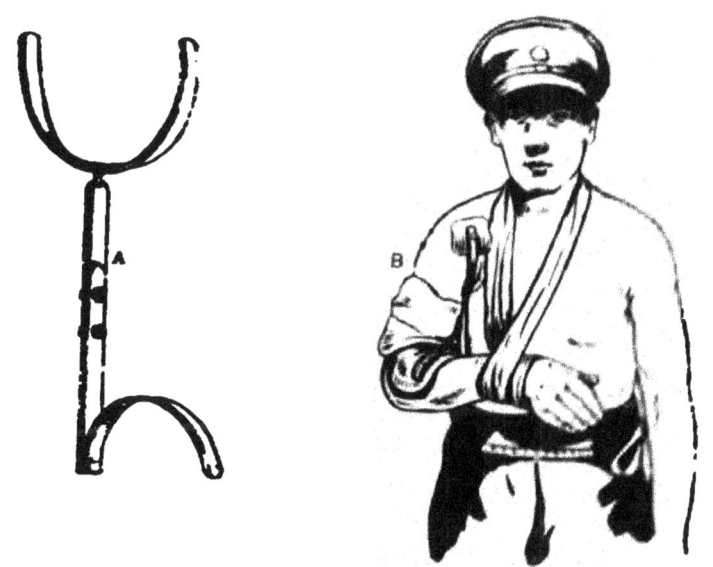

Fig. 11.—A, Depage's modified humerus splint. B, Applied for fracture of right humerus.

are other advantages possessed to the same degree by no other splints with which we are familiar."

52 TREATMENT OF WAR WOUNDS

Splints are thus "standardized." He urges, quite properly, I think, that they supplant plaster-of-Paris. I regret that space does not allow the reproduction of these cuts also.

For *extension* by means of *adhesive plaster* the following directions are taken from the Brit. Med. Jour., July 14, 1917:

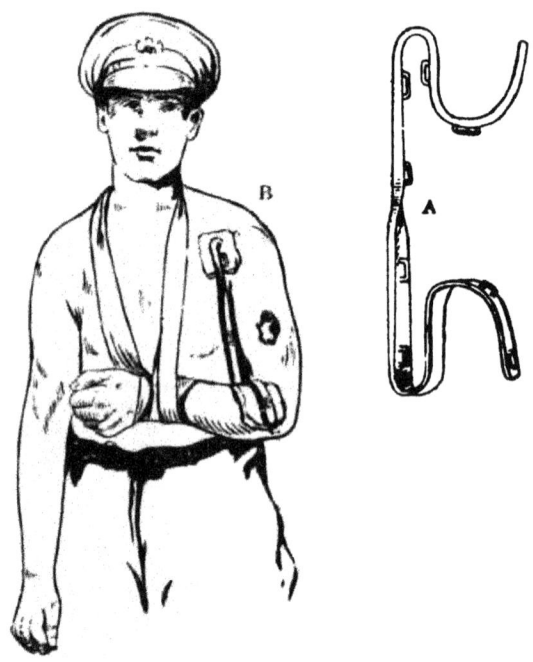

Fig. 12.—A, Extempore aluminum or strong wire splint for fracture of humerus. B, Applied for fracture of left humerus.

"Last August we published a note on a method of fixing extension to fractured limbs by the use of a glue adhesive, introduced by Major M. Sinclair, R.A.M.C., for use especially in the application of the extension to compound fractures of the lower

FRACTURES

limb. As we have received inquiries with regard to this, we have obtained information as to the formula

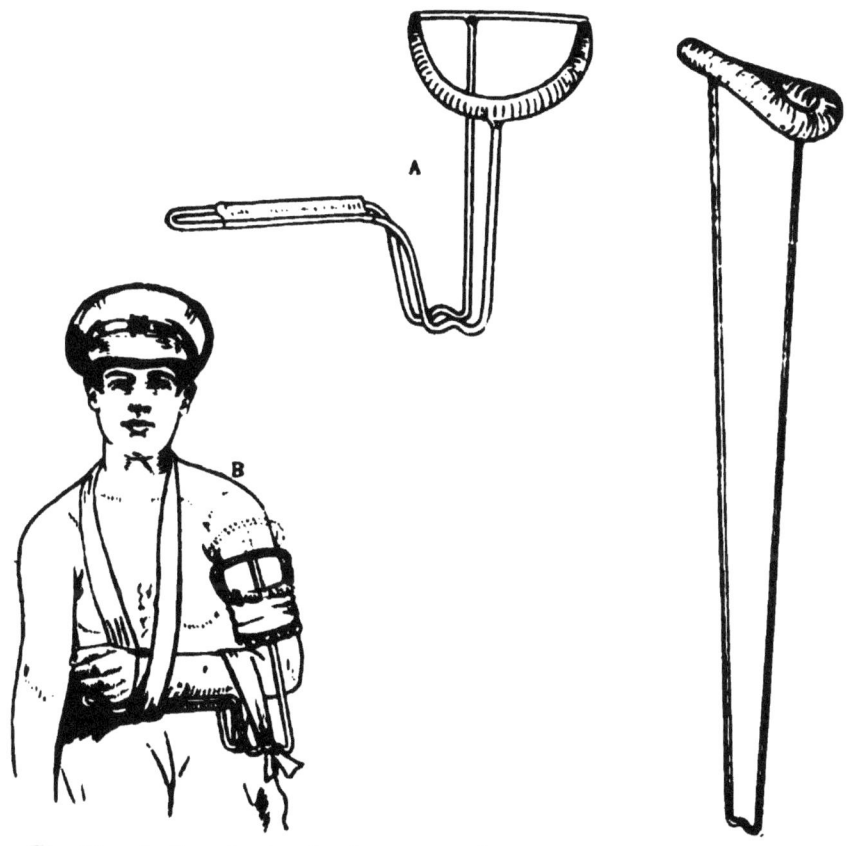

Fig. 13.—A, Jones' extension humerus splint. B, Applied for fracture of left humerus. The padded portion should be higher up in the axilla.

Fig. 14.—Thomas' knee splint.

at present used and the method of application. The formula in general use is as follows:

Ordinary glue	50 parts
Water	50 "
Glycerin	2 "
Calcium chlorid	2 "
Thymol	1 part

"The glycerin and calcium chlorid are both deliquescent and take up the perspiration, which keeps the glue from getting brittle, and, more important

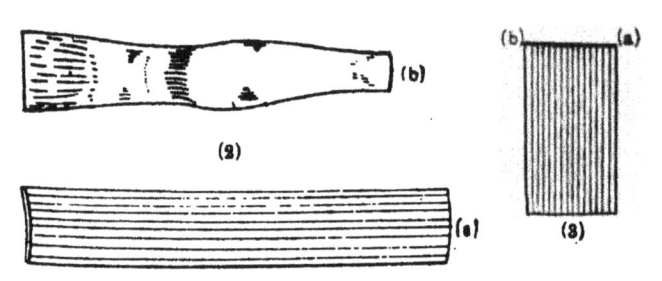

Fig. 15.—(2) The posterior supporting splint of Thomas' knee splint: (a) Gooch's splinting, 26" x 5"; (b) wooden ham splint; (c) Jones' metal fracture or gutter splint (padded with felt) is *not* illustrated. The largest sizes only should be used. (3) Short anterior thigh piece of Thomas' splint. The corners (a) for right and (b) for left thigh should be cut away.

still, allows perspiration to take place. This prevents the skin from getting sodden, in which condition bacteria may flourish and give rise to skin troubles. The thymol is added to prevent putrefaction and diminish smell. Every time the adhesive is heated the odour gets less and less. Experiments have proved that bacteria do not grow on this preparation. Air-tight tins which hold about a pound are filled and sterilized at 100° and placed in store. When required, the contents are melted in a water-bath, and set aside a few minutes to cool.

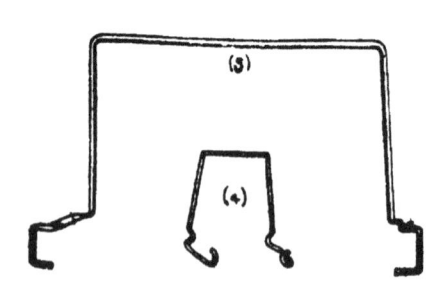

Fig. 16.—(4) Foot piece—strong wire. (5) Stretcher suspension bar.

"The adhesive is applied with the palm of the hand or a brush. The skin is washed with soap and sodium carbonate solution (four drachms to the pint) in order to remove fat, and when dry, the adhesive is applied *without* shaving the part. The area is covered evenly, and the ordinary four-ply gauze as it comes out of the packet applied, having roughly measured the requirements and gathered it in at the level of the wrist or ankle. An alternative method is to put on a length of 'Elastic cotton net bandage' (S. Maw) from knee to ankle, to glue it on the *outside*, and then to apply the gauze as above and bandage carefully with a thin bandage.

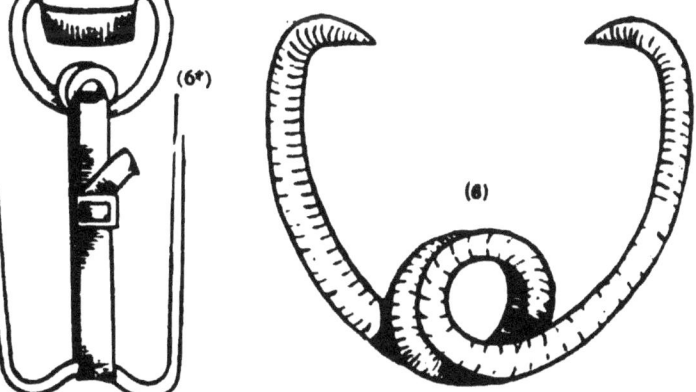

Fig. 17.—Tapson's heel clip (6) and its application (6*).

"The gauze, being spread out fan-shaped, adapts

Fig. 18.—Fracture of thigh put up in Thomas' splint.

mula gives an excellent adhesive which is a little more elastic:

    Isinglass..........................50 parts
    Glue.............................50 "
    Water............................50 "
    Calcium chlorid.................. 2
    Tannic acid......................12 "
    Thymol.......................... 1 part
    Glycerin......................... 2 parts"

Sir Robert Jones also considers gunshot injuries of *joints* and deprecates very many unwise *primary excisions of joints*, resulting so often in flail elbows,

FRACTURES

knees, and shoulders. Immediate excision of the

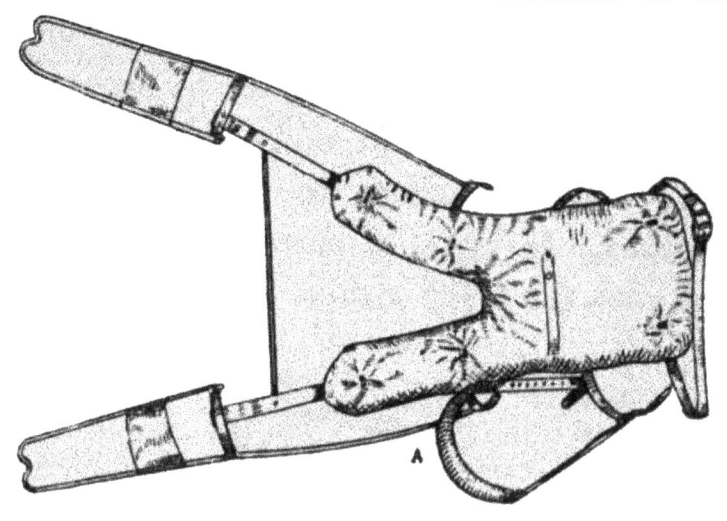

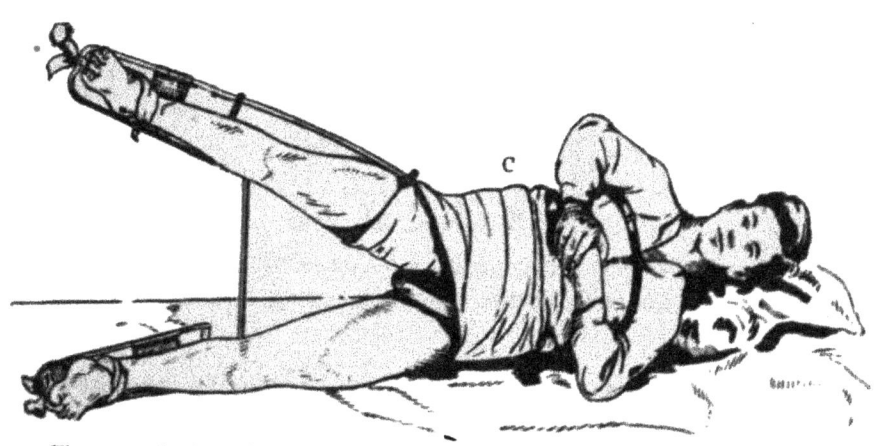

Fig. 19.—A, Jones' abduction frame for fracture of femur, when the accompanying wounds prevent the use of Thomas' splint outfit. These frames ought to be made with joints opposite the hip, so that they can be used for either side and can be "closed" for transport on a stretcher. C, To show the method of application. Temporary clove-hitch used around each ankle.

wound (not of the joint) has given results which are surprisingly good.

It is impossible to give anything like an adequate summary of this article. It should be read by every orthopedic surgeon, and in fact by *every* surgeon, in order that he may not make mistakes and deliver badly treated patients to the orthopedic central hospitals. It is most encouraging to learn that, even with the many serious and difficult cases which

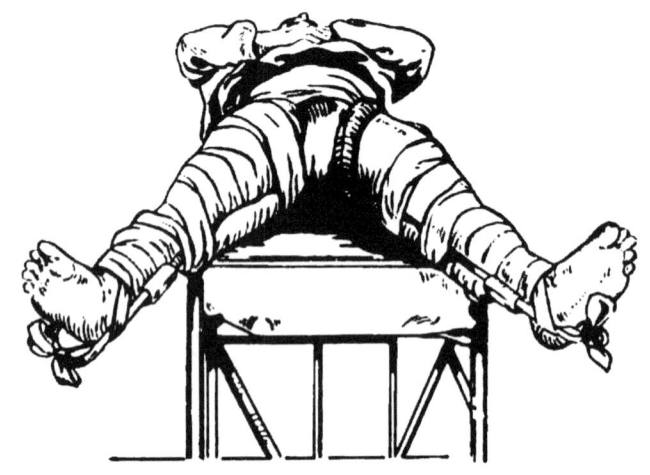

Fig. 20.—Jones' abduction frame applied for fracture of right femur. The extension strapping should reach high up on each limb.

Sir Robert receives, in the 16 orthopedic centers in the British Islands, containing nearly 15,000 wounded under his supervision, 75 per cent. have been returned to the army!

Chase gives a useful little hint as to plaster, viz.: Just before the cast is dry it may be coated with talcum powder well rubbed in. This makes a smooth

FRACTURES

surface, which can be washed, and on it the date and other memoranda may be written.

The "Balkan splint" (Fig. 21) is simple, useful, and

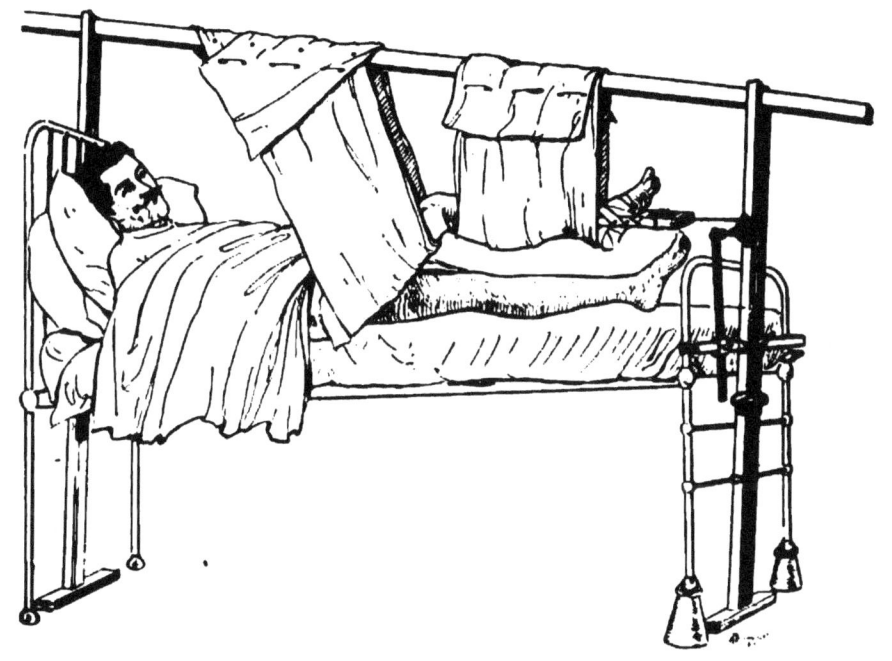

Fig. 21.—Balkan splint as used at the American Ambulance, Neuilly-sur-Seine, Paris, France. (Crile, in Annals of Surgery, July, 1915. Attributed to Lt. Col. Miles by Sir Geo. H. Makins, Brit. Med. Jour., June 16, 1917.)

widely employed in hospitals, but it is not adapted for transportation.

Crile insists rightly upon the value of morphin for men suffering severely, whether in hospitals or during transportation. It should be given early and usually a half-grain for the first dose. After the second Bull Run, when a train of over 100 ambulances carrying the wounded to Washington, after they had been lying for three days uncared for and undressed, halted in the night at Centreville, I found the three most needed things were drinking water, hot soup, and morphin. On the other hand, too much morphin is as bad as too little, especially in abdominal cases.

BIBLIOGRAPHY OF SOME IMPORTANT BOOKS AND PAPERS ON MILITARY ORTHOPEDICS

Jones: Injuries to Joints.
Jones: Notes on Military Orthopedics.
Mayer: Orthopedic Treatment of Gunshot Injuries, W. B. Saunders Company, 1918.
Benisty: "The Clinical Forms of Nerve Lesions," University of London Press, London.
Bensity: The Treatment and Repair of Nerve Lesions.
Leriche: The Treatment of Fractures (Fractures involving Joints).
Leriche: The Treatment of Fractures (Fractures of the Shaft).
Broca: The After-effects of Wounds of the Bones and Joints.
Aitken: "The Treatment of Gunshot Fractures," Brit. Med. Jour., August 12, 1916.
Aitken: "Orthopedic Methods in Military Surgery," Trans. Med. Soc. London, vol. xl.
Souttar: "Some Points Arising in Nerve Injuries," Brit. Med. Jour., December 22, 1917.
Renfrew White: "Fifty Cases of Injury to Peripheral Nerves," Brit. Jour. Surg., April, 1917.
Naughton Dunn: "Treatment of Lesions of Musculo-spiral Nerve in Military Surgery," to be published in Amer. Jour. Orthop. Surg., 1918.

Stiles: "Operative Treatment of Nerve Injuries," to be published in Amer. Jour. Orthop. Surg., 1918.

Gray: "Early Treatment of Gunshot Wounds of the Knee-joint," Brit. Med. Jour., September 1, 1917.

Barling: "Treatment of Gunshot Wounds of the Knee-Joint," Brit. Med. Jour., September 1, 1917.

Cook: "Gunshot Wounds of the Joint: Their Pathology and Treatment," Lancet, May 12, 1917.

Little: "Modern Artificial Limbs and their Influence upon Methods of Amputation," Brit. Med. Jour., October 27, 1917.

NEW WEAPONS

New weapons have caused a new type of wounds. At first there were many bullet wounds, then shrapnel wounds outnumbered those caused by the rifle, and now the high explosive shell is the chief weapon.

In the wounded from Verdun Captain W. E. Lee tells me that wounds by bullets and shells were noted in the hospitals in the proportion of 15 to 85.

Hand grenades thrown by the soldier and high explosive bombs dropped from airplanes are also very constantly employed and cause severe lacerations.

Artillery has leaped into new and dominating importance. These shells, all surgeons agree, produce terrible and wide-spread mutilations.

Fig. 22 (which I owe to the kindness of Captain W. Estell Lee) shows the shape of three shell fragments. It is no wonder that such missiles should produce the most frightfully lacerated wounds, tearing the tissues almost inconceivably.

Fragments of the shells not only may lodge, but also in most cases carry with them deep into the tissues, in the majority of wounds, bits of dirty cloth-

NEW WEAPONS

ing, skin, and other foreign bodies, all heavily infected. Diligent search must be made for such foci of infection at the very first opportunity for a thor-

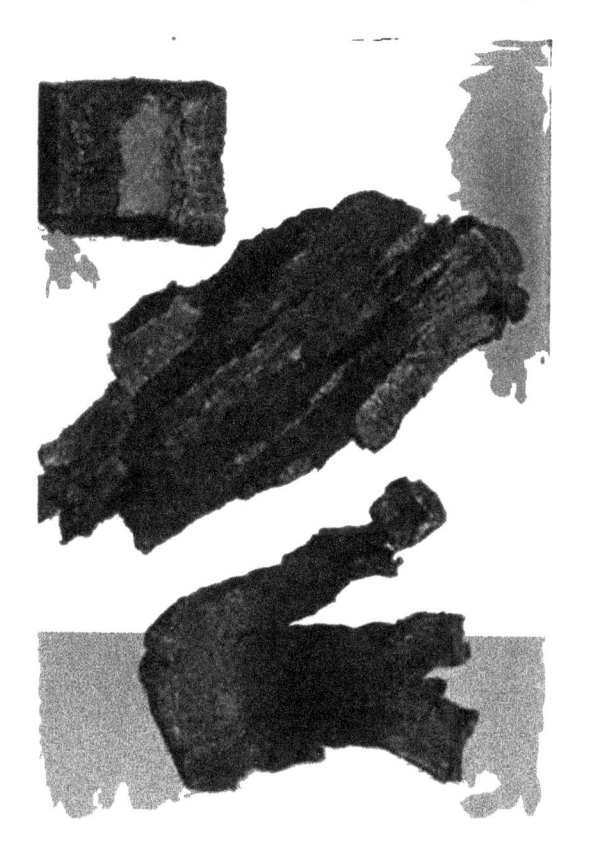

Fig. 22.—Fragments of a shell to indicate what terrible lacerations they must cause (courtesy of Capt. W. Estell Lee).

ough dressing, or deep and wide-spread infection is sure to follow.

Fig. 23 (which I also owe to Captain Lee) shows (B) a piece of clothing driven deep into the flesh by a fragment of shell (A). Observe how nearly the bit of clothing approximates to the shape and size of the shell-fragment almost as if it had been "punched out" by a machine. Captain Lee tells me that now,

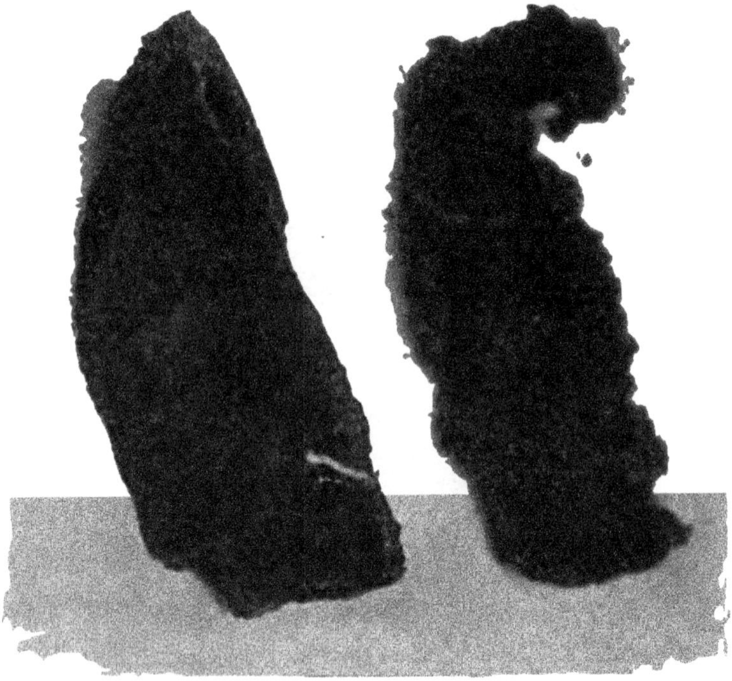

A B

Fig. 23.—A, Fragment of shell; B, piece of clothing "punched out" by the fragment of shell and carried deep into the tissues (courtesy of Capt. W. Estell Lee).

before attempting to remove a bit of cloth, it is the rule to measure exactly the size and shape of the hole in the clothing and to compare with this the bit of clothing removed. The surgeon can thus assure himself whether he has removed *all* of the indriven piece of clothing or should continue his search.

Crile* has described a new secondary missile— mud. "A high explosive shell would dive into the mud and throw the mud with such tremendous velocity that it would actually cause a penetration of the skin; and through that hole a vast amount of mud would be forced, producing a very bad type of wound, and in some instances death."

It must not be forgotten that these modern bullets and fragments of high explosive shells produce grave destruction of tissue not merely in the track of the missile, but that the tissues at varying distances all around and beyond the wounds are devitalized. This destruction is often not recognizable by the eye or touch until some time has passed. Bowlby, quoted by Moynihan,† has shown that a kidney wounded in its lower pole presented to the naked eye a normal appearance at its upper end, but the microscope showed that the tubules in that part were disorganized.

The testimony as to the wide devitalizing and even pulpifying force of high velocity missiles seems to be well established. Thus Archibald and Gamlen and Smith (*vide* p. 182) show how the brain and the mus-

* Jour. Amer. Med. Assoc., November 3, 1917, p. 1539.
† Brit. Med. Jour., March 4, 1916.

cles may be pulpified. The former states that the muscles "may be pulped for 1 to 3 inches" away from the track. "The explosive force, radiated laterally, not only devitalizes the tissues (so that often one can wipe off muscle tissue with a swab), but also separates them as one might fluff out a feather-duster by blowing into it. The same force drives into the recesses, momentarily formed, infected foreign bodies of all sorts.

On the other hand, Bashford,* by a most painstaking examination of wounds of the kidney, liver, spleen, etc., found that microscopically there was no evidence of severe vibratory effects at a distance from the track of the missile. He warns, therefore, against *too* wide excision. Yet the cases above quoted seem to show that in some cases at least the damage done *is* wide-spread. Of the two extremes, too wide excision is less dangerous than too restricted excision.

This wide-spread devitalizing of the tissues has led to the common-sense practice, especially urged by Carrel, after primary thorough mechanical cleansing and disinfection, of excision of the tissues surrounding the wound itself instead of allowing them to undergo gradual necrosis and serve as an excellent nidus for infection.

* Brit. Jour. Surg., 1917, iv, 433.

Shells and shrapnel also frequently cause *multiple* wounds. The fragments of a shattered bone act as additional secondary projectiles and further enlarge the area of destruction. Chase* says that "multiple wounds are the rule. . . . Thirty, forty, or fifty wounds from the explosion of a shell close by are not particularly rare." He then describes one stretcher-bearer who had "well over one hundred wounds. We picked out pieces of shell, newspaper, clothing, and gravel for days afterward." Fortunately, no one of the wounds was serious, and in the course of a month he was ready for furlough.

Colonel Dercle, of the French Medical Service, so admired by all of us for his fortitude and his bonhomie, has visited America with Director General Goodwin already mentioned. He has survived 97 simultaneous wounds. His life long held by a thread, but he finally recovered with, it is true, a halting gait, but there was no "halting" in his fervid, contagious patriotism.

Multiple wounds may profoundly modify the decision as to operation.

All these complicating conditions complicate also the treatment. But the chief outstanding fact is virulent and all-pervading infection.

*Annals of Surgery, July, 1917.

The soil of Belgium and France has been cultivated for over twenty centuries, since even before the days of Cæsar's Gallic War, when he conquered and praised the *brave Belgians.* The fields have been roamed over by cattle, horses, swine, and other animals, including man himself; the soil has been manured thousands of times, and so is deeply and thoroughly impregnated with fecal bacteria in addition to the ordinary pyogenic bacteria.

The soldiers have lived in trenches for months, begrimed and bedaubed with mud, without suitable facilities for bathing and change of under and outer clothing, especially in the early days of the war. It was not uncommon at that period for a man to be unable to change even his trousers for weeks. When, therefore, a missile carried into the wound a piece of dirty, mud-impregnated skin, coat, trousers, underclothing, or socks, or when a large lacerated wound was in contact with the long-soiled clothing, and the wounded man would perhaps he on the ground uncared for for hours or days, it was no wonder that violent infection from pyogenic organisms followed, and that the bacteria of tetanus and gas gangrene ran riot.

Carrel[*] has observed that when a wound was ex-

[*] Bull. Acad. Méd., lxxiv, No. 40, and Brit. Med. Jour., Oct. 23, 1915.

amined bacteriologically as early as six hours after it had been inflicted, there was found a varied flora of both aërobic and anaërobic bacteria, but that they were few in number, and localized chiefly around the missile or a bit of clothing, etc., without as yet spreading far and wide into the tissues. Twenty-four hours later, however, the bacteria were found everywhere, and were too numerous to count. Moreover, as Wright has pointed out, when there has been delay in dressing a wound, the dried blood sealing the wound creates an almost ideal condition for the growth of the deadly anaërobic bacteria of tetanus and gas gangrene. (*Vide infra,* Tissier's observation, p. 162.) It is no wonder then that experience has shown that excision of this damaged and heavily infected tissue is one of the prime factors in the treatment of the badly wounded.

Bowlby (*loc. cit.*) points out that "if a badly wounded man cannot be rescued and brought into the field ambulance until after the lapse of twenty-four or thirty-six hours, the wound is often already so badly infected and the patient himself is in so toxic a state that surgical treatment has but little chance. It may be said truly that the most important alteration in treatment since the early days of the war is that excision of damaged tissue has become the routine method, and that the earlier it is carried out, the more likely it is to be successful."

Whatever other treatment surgeons may advocate, they all unite now in this advice: (1) Remove all foreign bodies, especially clothing, the chief carrier of tetanus and gas-gangrene infection; and (2) "ruthless excision," all in one piece, if possible, with care not to reinfect the new raw surface. Of course, there are wounds which cannot be ruthlessly excised for anatomic reasons, *e. g.*, when this would mean excision of large vessels, opening of the pleural or the peritoneal cavity, or would require so extensive removal of tissue as to impair too seriously the function of the part, etc. Common sense must over-ride even dogmatic rules in such cases. But life, it must be remembered, is superior to the preservation of function, valuable as the latter may be.

Haycroft[*] reports the results of treating 116 cases by *soap and water and primary suture*. The experiment was suggested to him by Colonel Cuthbert Wallace. The soap solution was made of one part of sapo durus cut into shavings and dissolved in 20 parts of hot boiled water. When used, it is diluted with an equal quantity of hot water, making it 1 : 40. "Success depends—(1) on getting cases *within a few*

[*] Brit. Med. Jour., January 19, 1918.

hours, before infective processes have spread far . . .
(2) on the thorough removal of dead or grossly damaged tissue" and (3) on the removal of all foreign bodies.

The technic is as follows: The track of the wound is laid open if practicable, followed by complete excision of the wound, thus leaving an aseptic surface. This is thoroughly swabbed out with the soap solution. Muscles and fasciæ are closed by catgut, and the skin sutured. When not practicable to lay open the entire wound, it is reached partly from each end. If any portion cannot be excised, it is well rubbed with gauze and soap. If a dead space is left after suture, a very small split rubber tube is inserted and left for twenty-four to forty-eight hours. He points out that "the tissues themselves are able to deal successfully with any [slight] infection which is left behind." Sometimes a local reaction follows for two or three days but "subsides as the tissues gain the upper hand."

A most important point is that no case so treated should be evacuated for at least a week, first, because any movement is most prejudicial, and secondly, in case of a sharp reaction, no new surgeon can decide on what is to be done so well as the original operator.

Two objections are mentioned: (1) The soap makes

instruments slippery, and (2) the method takes so much time that it is impracticable during a period of severe pressure.

Results of 98 cases completely observed showed 91 healed and 7 failed. Of 38 compound fractures, 33 healed and 2 failed. Of compound fractures of the femur, there were only 3 cases, of which 2 were successful. Evidently, as he says, one cannot draw reliable conclusions from so small a number.

Amputations were completely closed with a very small split drainage-tube at one corner for twenty-four hours.

Penetrating wounds of the *knee-joint* were completely excised down to the synovial membrane; the joint well irrigated with the soap solution, and the wound closed in layers.

It will be observed that the whole method is based on the wounds being only superficially infected, *i. e.*, can be dressed within a very few hours, and the technic is of the strictest aseptic procedures.

Could there possibly be stronger reasons for urging that every wounded man, if it is at all possible, should obtain thorough care during the very first golden hours, when efficient treatment would save his life? Military conditions may, and too often do, prevent this early dressing, but this, above all other factors for recovery, should be the aim both of the surgeon and the commander, for so human lives are saved and armies are less depleted by death and disability.

During the Civil War maggots were very common in the summer. Even mosquito netting on a frame several inches high to expose the wound to air and sunlight did not prevent their presence. The fly would perch on the frame, and with more than the accuracy of the modern aviator, drop her eggs on to the wound. The resulting maggots were certainly disgusting, but, so far as I ever observed, they did no harm.

Crile now says[*] that, on the contrary, they actually do good! "In the wounded who lie out in 'No Man's Land' for two or five or ten days, it has been found that the wounds that have done best are those that contain maggots. The reason for this is that there is devitalized tissue; the maggots live on this devitalized tissue, and if they destroy that tissue, they do in time what the surgical operation does."

This would probably be especially true in cases of infection from the bacillus of gas gangrene.

In the navy, on the contrary, where the factor of infected soil is not present, "sailors with the most severe type of wounds, ragged, irregular, with uneven

[*] Jour. Amer. Med. Assoc., November 3, 1917, 1540.

surface, produced by herniated muscles and retracted, severed fibers, usually recovered quickly."*

Moreover, in the terrible but magnificent retreat from the Aisne to the Marne, many, and in some cases almost every man was exhausted to the last degree mentally as well as physically. Crile† has given a wonderful picture of the exhaustion of these patients, who practically slept while they marched, and slept through painful dressings or even during operations. The nervous strain to which the men are subjected in the trenches impairs greatly their ability to withstand the almost malignant infection which invades the great gaping wounds.

Goodwin‡ gives this good advice as to the care of patients who have been received from the front: Always remove the dressing applied at the front, for it is almost sure to be contaminated. Even if this has not occurred, infection is likely to follow from the fact that the dressing has been applied over a contaminated skin, which there may have been no opportunity of cleansing. The surgeon and assistants should always wear rubber gloves and gowns, changing them as required. Always remove a tourniquet

* Jour. Amer. Med. Assoc., May 22, 1915, p. 1765.
† Military Surgeon, September, 1917, p. 279.
‡ Mechanistic View of War and Peace, Macmillan, 1916.

if one has been used. Very likely it has been applied too tightly, and even if not, the subsequent swelling has made it too tight.

Early experiences in the war demonstrated the fact that both antisepsis and asepsis as heretofore practised had been vanquished by Mars. Each was tried and each failed. It was even proclaimed that Lister's work went for naught. Now, however, antisepsis and asepsis (in its proper place) have come into their own again, and Lister is still the apostle of good tidings. The reasons are plain: First, we did not then possess sufficiently effective antiseptics, such as modern research has now given us; second, we were not masters of an effective and successful technic. We owe these especially to two men—Dakin and Carrel—who have wrought a marvelous revolution.

Lister taught us, above all, how to *prevent* infection; Dakin and Carrel, following Lister's principles, have taught us how to *conquer* even rampant infection. For nearly half a century we surgeons have been fighting firmly intrenched infection, but always in vain. It required the stern stimulus of war to enable us to win the victory. Prevention and cure both are now ours.

Among several newer antiseptics as to which there are rather conflicting reports, "*flavine*" (or, as it is better called, "*acriflavine*") and "*proflavine*" have their friends and enemies. The experimental evidence *in vitro* on the whole seems to be possibly adverse, but the clinical evidence *in vivo*, certainly the most important, I judge is distinctly in their favor.

Mercurophen is still in the experimental stage.

Four principal methods of treatment have been developed by the surgical experiences of the war.

First, and most important, that known as the *Carrel-Dakin* method.

Second, the *dichloramin-T* treatment. This is an outgrowth of experience with the first Dakin solution of the hypochlorite of soda. Dakin has substituted the dichloramin salt, twice as rich in chlorin, for the chloramin-T which he first used. As I shall indicate, this new preparation in some important respects seems to be better than his first hypochlorite of soda. It is, however, only a change in one portion of Carrel's method. The rest of Carrel's technic, the wide excision* of all damaged tissue; the later

---

* I am told that the term "excision-revision" is in frequent use in France to indicate this procedure. I must enter an earnest protest against such wretched English. "Revision" is not only unnecessary, but confuses the reader. When I first saw the term I was totally at a loss to know what the compound phrase meant. It had to be explained to me.

substitution of the paste dressing; the constant bacteriologic testing of the degree of sterilization; and incidentally du Noüy's ingenious "curve of healing" —are quite as important as the particular chlorin salt employed.

Dakin deserves the greatest credit for his discovery, as one may well call it, that the chlorin preparations are the best antiseptics for wounds. Not only do they attack and destroy the bacteria without injuring the tissue cells, if used in proper dilution, but they dissolve and carry away devitalized and necrotic tissue—a matter of the greatest importance, especially in cases infected with the gas-producing bacilli. His dichloramin-T may easily prove to be an improvement over the chloramin-T.

Third, the "*Bipp*" treatment, introduced by Rutherford Morison, of Newcastle-on-Tyne, and

Fourth, Sir Almroth Wright's Hypertonic Salt Solution and Gray's modification—the salt-pack. This last has had a certain vogue but, if I may judge by reading and the reports of friends in the British and American troops in France, is not growing in favor. As I must crowd so much into so little space I am compelled to omit this method.

A very interesting paper by Donaldson and Joyce[*]

[*] Lancet, September 22, 1917.

gives some curious facts as to a bacillus which they temporarily have named the "Reading bacillus," from the location of their hospital. It produces a characteristic foul odor in wounds treated by the salt-pack. Experiments seemed to show that those wounds improved which developed this bad smell and those which did not develop it did not improve. So they deliberately infected wounds not having this odor and not doing well with this bacillus and reported immediate improvement. The method is too new to have had its real value as yet determined.

The controversy over the Carrel-Dakin treatment has not always been carried on with that calmness of spirit and scientifically cool and balanced judgment which is the only proper attitude. He has even been sneered at as a mere "laboratory man," as if that were a reproach! Yet for years his "laboratory work" on animals has been actively clinical, and for the last three years his intensive clinical work at Compiègne has been unsurpassed. I shall quote the opinions of only a few whose opportunities and judgment seem to me most worthy of consideration. A personal visit to Carrel at the War Demonstration Hospital of the Rockefeller Institute in New York convinced me—if I needed any conviction—that the results were the best evidence of the merits of the method.

The two most important witnesses are unquestionably Professor Wm. H. Welch and Professor Depage.

The testimony of Professor Wm. H. Welch, of Johns Hopkins,* is most valuable because of his eminence as a pathologist and as a broad-minded philosophic observer.

Dr. Welch's Testimony.—After a visit to Compiègne,—not a casual visit, but one during which he studied the method and the smears "day by day,"— Welch says:

"There can be no question that Carrel deserves the credit—and a very considerable credit this is—of recalling the attention of surgeons to the possibility of the sterilization of infected wounds by chemical means. The idea is, of course, not new, but is the original Listerian one. That the Carrel-Dakin procedure actually accomplishes such sterilization sufficiently for surgical purposes is quite conclusively demonstrated, and whatever changes be made in his technic as the result of further experiences, he will deserve the credit of reapplying a great surgical principle of wound treatment, which had been practically abandoned."

. . . . "It was fascinating to watch [by the microscope] the reduction, often astonishingly rapid, at other times slower, of these bacteria under irrigation by the Dakin fluid. It was a quite novel thing

* Jour. Amer. Med. Assoc., December 8, 1917.

to find the bacteriologist occupying this relation to the surgeon and telling him when the wound could be safely closed. The cicatrization after closure under this bacterial control was amazingly rapid." . . .

"I see no conflict with the teachings of surgical pathology in Carrel's work. . . . Experience with the Carrel method proves conclusively that the destruction of these surface bacteria, without injury to the body tissues, is of primary importance. So many who discuss this question seem to lose sight of the fact that a great principle is really involved, viz., that of the sterilization of wounds by chemical methods without damage to cells, and the influence of such sterilization on the repair of wounds. Carrel's work is fundamental on this point." . . . The actual results are quite unequaled, as Almroth Wright himself told me, and as so many have testified."

Depage has a hospital of 800 beds at La Panne, Belgium, within a few kilometers of the trenches. After studying the Carrel-Dakin method at Compiègne he has adopted it and practised it with great success. "Imitation is the sincerest flattery."

Colonel G. Barling* first studied Carrel's method at Compiègne, then in Tuffier's wards, in J. P. Hutchinson's wards at the American Ambulance, in Chut-

* Brit. Jour. Surg., 1917, v, 116.

ro's wards, all three in Paris, and finally in his own wards in Rouen. At Compiègne he says, "I felt that I was in the presence of successful Wound Treatment, *such as I had not seen approached by any other method*," and after using it in his own wards he concludes: "We have attained such a measure of success as I have not seen secured by other methods and I anticipate that further experience will give still better results."

See also Professor W. S. Halsted's letter, p. 252.

Personally, I have seen none of these methods used. I can judge only by the published results. "By their fruits ye shall know them." Judging by this standard, I am forced to conclude that one method—that of Carrel and Dakin—has shown results much superior to the others. If I am asked to give the reason, I need only quote the following paragraphs, describing what Dr. C. L. Gibson, of New York,* saw at La Panne, Belgium, where the method is strictly and efficiently carried out:

"Dr. Depage greeted me by saying that he had 80 compound fractures all grouped in one ward and that not one was suppurating. He kindly devoted a whole forenoon to their demonstration, and I had an oppor-

* General Bulletin, Society of the New York Hospital, March 27, 1917.

tunity to see every one of these 80 cases, even to the smallest details. None of the dressings were touched till I had an opportunity to see them and estimate the amount and nature of the discharge contained on them. I had an opportunity also to see the bacterial chart of every one of these cases, see a number of these cases 'closed,' and in some cases observe their condition and final healing. I was able not only to corroborate Dr. Depage's statement that not one of these compound fractures was suppurating, but could affirm, in addition, that I failed to see a single drop of pus in any one of these cases. When one remembers that these wounds offer the maximum possibilities, particularly the shell wounds, with terrific mangling of the tissues, extensive splintering of bone, harboring many and diverse forms of projectiles and foreign bodies, necessarily all primarily infected,—in other words, the worst possible imaginable wounds,— the result is something one must know for oneself to appreciate.

"These wounds heal in a manner that is simply indescribable. One has to see the behavior of these sutured wounds oneself to realize what happens. They heal with no more reaction from their appearance and manifestations than would be given by a wound which has been sutured on a cadaver—total absence of reaction, pain, swelling, redness, and even of infiltration around the wound edges. Dr. Dchelly, of Havre, tells me that he has closed 400 of these wounds with only six failures to obtain perfect primary union. Of these six mishaps, none was of any importance, and in some of these Dehelly said the fault was probably due to his failure to await complete sterilization, as evidenced by the bacterial count."

I have never yet seen any report of 80 cases of compound fracture of the thigh without a drop of pus when treated by any other method. When myself in active practice, I should have been more than gratified had I realized such a result, even in the best of conditions and in civil life, where infection is far more easily dealt with.

Lee and Furness[*] state that whereas their mortality (with the Carrel-Dakin method) was 4.6 per cent. in 1915, in 1916 it had been reduced to 1.9 per cent., *i. e.*, much below one-half of the mortality in 1915. This they attribute largely to the fact that in 1915 it was not at all uncommon for men only to reach efficient surgical aid from five to seven days after being wounded, whereas in 1916 the average was only one and one-half hours. In 1916 immediate excision of all devitalized tissue and removal of the foreign body within three hours was constantly

[*] Captain W. E. Lee, M.R.C., U.S.A., and Captain W. H. Furness, M.R.C., U.S.A., "The Treatment of Infectious and Infected Wounds," to appear in the "Military Surgeon" early in 1918.

accomplished. Another element contributing to these better results (and largely depending on the early arrival of the wounded where they could be efficiently treated) was this. In the battle in the Champagne (1915) 80 per cent. of the cases were infected with the gas gangrene organisms in the cultures, and 60 per cent. had clinical symptoms. In the battle of the Somme (1916) only 20 per cent. showed in cultures the organisms of gas gangrene and only 5 per cent. developed clinical symptoms of the disease. In 1915 the mortality was 4.6%; in 1916 only 1.9%.

Tuffier alleges that 80 per cent. of all amputations are due to infection. If we can now conquer infection, most of these mutilations will probably be avoided.

What an immense boon this will be to the soldiers, and therefore to the community, by enabling them, even if only partly, to earn their daily bread, is most evident. The military commanders will be equally gratified by the return to their commands of many of the wounded who otherwise would have been returned to civil life in this mutilated condition or have been carried to the cemetery.

It is but fair to state that independently in the British Medical Journal, July 24, 1915, p. 129, Lorrain Smith, Drennan, Rettie, and Campbell, of the Department of Pathology in the University of Edinburgh, published their "Experimental Observations on the Antiseptic Action of Hypochlorous Acid and its Application to Wound Treatment." They devised two forms of its use—a powder which they named *Eupad*, and a solution which they named *Eusol*. Eupad consisted of equal weights of finely ground bleaching powder (chlorid of lime) and of boric acid. Eusol was standardized at 0.5 per cent. of hypochlorous acid. Both of these preparations have been much used with good results, but, on the whole, they do not seem to have been so satisfactory or at least have not gained the same wide-spread repute as Dakin's fluid.

THE CARREL-DAKIN METHOD

The method requires special training. To provide this training the Rockefeller Foundation in 1917 erected a War Demonstration Hospital on the grounds of the Rockefeller Institute in New York, and for a number of months had the personal services of Carrel for the instruction of surgeons in the military service of the country.

A very common and possibly the general impression as to Carrel's method is that it consists chiefly—or as some even appear to think, solely—in the application of Dakin's solution to the wound by means of a lot of tubes. This was my own impression at first. This is only a part of his method, though a very important part. But it is far more than that, as has been pointed out by Welch (p. 79) and by Colonel W. C. Borden,* who writes: "Carrel's treatment of infected wounds is as definitely worked out as is the aseptic technic of a modern operating room, and constitutes a *surgical method*, not merely the application of an *antiseptic agent*."

* Internat. Jour. Surg. (to appear early in 1918).

Carrel's publications are in part responsible for this, as the chief prominence is given to his means of applying Dakin's solution. But quite as important is his insistence on the surgical *removal of all foreign bodies and of the infected walls immediately lining the track of the missile, and of all the devitalized and necrotic tissues surrounding this track.* Dakin's solution then attacks the bacteria and also the necrotic, devitalized tissues which may have escaped the knife, and chemically sterilizes the wound. Then a *chloramin paste* (p. 93) is substituted for the hypochlorite solution. The wound is closed only when the constantly made bacterial count—another important innovation—shows the wound to be "surgically sterile."

Dakin's Hypochlorite Solution.—*Definition.*—Dakin's solution is a solution of sodium hypochlorite (NaOCl), which contains not less than 0.4 per cent. nor more than 0.5 per cent. sodium hypochlorite; and which is not alkaline to powdered phenolphthalein but is alkaline to alcoholic solution of phenolphthalein. If the percentage of sodium hypochlorite is less than 0.4 per cent., the antiseptic power of the solution is too low; if greater than 0.5 per cent., the solution is irritating. If the solution is alkaline to powdered phenolphthalein, the solution is irritating;

if the solution is acid to alcoholic solution of phenolphthalein, the solution is unstable.

[McCartney and Mewburn,* after painstaking investigation, fix 0.485 as the optimum, *i. e.*, best percentage.—K.]

Measure 10 c.c. of Dakin's solution, using a bulb pipet, into a beaker or Erlenmeyer flask containing about 50 to 100 c.c. of tap-water. The disappearance of color is most easily observed when the volume of fluid in the vessel is between 50 and 100 c.c.

Add 5 c.c. of a 10 per cent. potassium (or sodium) iodid solution and 5 c.c. of glacial acetic acid. Then run decinormal thiosulphate solution into the flask from a buret until the decolorization of the solution is complete. The flask with the contents should be vigorously agitated during the titration.

The number of cubic centimeters decinormal thiosulphate required to decolorize the solution, multiplied by the factor 0.0372, gives the percentage of sodium hypochlorite. For example:

12.10 c.c. × 0.0372 = 0.45 per cent.
13.43 c.c. × 0.0372 = 0.50 per cent.

The following definition and methods are those taught at the War Demonstration Hospital of the Rockefeller Institute:

* Brit. Med. Jour., February 9, 1918.

Tests for Alkalinity.—Test with powdered phenolphthalein: A few crystals of powdered phenolphthalein are dropped on the surface of about 5 c.c. of the solution to be tested and the solution vigorously shaken. Dakin's solution should remain entirely colorless. If there is any red color, the solution is too alkaline and must either be discarded or the excess alkalinity neutralized.

Test with alcoholic solution of phenolphthalein: About half a cubic centimeter of alcoholic solution of phenolphthalein (1 per cent.) is squirted from a dropper into about 5 c.c. of the solution to be tested, in a test-tube. The solution should show a red color which will soon disappear. If there is not at least a momentary flash of red color, the solution has so low an alkalinity that its hypochlorite content will rapidly diminish.

(*Note: It is important to remember that the tests of Dakin's solution for alkalinity and for strength of sodium hypochlorite are entirely independent, but equally important.*)

Preparation.—Dakin's solution may be satisfactorily prepared in any one of several ways:

First: By the electrolysis of a sodium chlorid solution. This method gives a satisfactory product, but requires apparatus and electric current that are not always available. Dakin has prepared a convenient apparatus for use on board ship.*

*Dakin, H. D., and Dunham, E. K.: Handbook of Antiseptics.

Second: By the action of chlorin on sodium carbonate. This simple method has hitherto been practically unavailable because of the difficulty of measuring liquid chlorin. This disadvantage has recently been overcome, and the method has proved entirely satisfactory.

Third: By the double decomposition of calcium hypochlorite and sodium carbonate. This method, the one first used by Dakin, because of the ease of obtaining the necessary chemicals, has been the most available one. The alkalinity of the solution, after the precipitation of the calcium as carbonate, may be neutralized either by the addition of boric acid (Dakin) or as described below.

Preparation from Chlorin and Sodium Carbonate.[*]—A solution is prepared containing 14 grams of dry sodium carbonate per liter (=16.6 grams monohydrate or 38 grams washing soda), a measured quantity, 4.8 grams per liter (or about 1600 c.c.) of chlorin gas is allowed to run into the solution. Chlorin may be obtained in liquid form in steel cylinders, and is easily measured by a chlorin meter manufactured for the purpose. This is a stable, economical, and convenient source of chlorin. Ten c.c. of the solution is then titrated. If the solution is too strong, it should be diluted to 0.5 per cent. NaOCl with 1 per cent. sodium carbonate, which serves to correct the unduly diminished alkalinity

[*] G. E. Cullen and J. H. Austin, Proc. Soc. Exp. Biol. and Med., December 19, 1917.

caused by the excess of chlorin introduced into the solution. However, the designated amount of carbonate is planned to give, at a concentration of 0.5 per cent. NaOCl, the minimum degree of alkalinity consistent with stability, and if chlorin has been introduced in such excess that the titer exceeds the desired by more than 3 or 4 c.c. of N/10 thiosulphate, or if the solution fails to give a momentary flash of color with *alcoholic solution of phenolphthalein*, it should be rejected. The solution must, of course, show no color with powdered phenolphthalein. The solution should be titrated for hypochlorite concentration every twenty-four or forty-eight hours.

Preparation from Bleaching Powder and Sodium Carbonate.—One hundred and forty grams of *dry* sodium carbonate (Na_2CO_3) or 400 grams of the crystallized salt (washing soda) are dissolved in 10 liters of tap water, and 200 grams of bleaching powder, containing 24 to 28 per cent. of "available chlorin," are added. The mixture is very thoroughly shaken, both to make good contact and to render the precipitated calcium carbonate granular and promote its settling. It is then allowed to stand quietly, and after half an hour the clear liquid is siphoned off from the precipitate and filtered through a cotton plug or paper. Forty grams of boric acid are added to the clear filtrate, and the resulting solution is ready for use. The boric acid must not be added before filtering but only afterward. The exact strength should be determined from time to time. It is important that the solution should not be stronger than 0.5 per cent. sodium hypochlorite or irritation of the skin may be frequent. On the other hand, it should not be less than 0.4 per cent. or its germicidal action is materially diminished. The solution should also be tested for neutrality by adding a little of it to a trace of solid phenolphthalein suspended in water. No red color indicating free alkali should develop, or else more boric acid must be added; this is, however, rarely necessary with the above proportions. The solution should not be kept longer than one week.

A *stronger solution* may be prepared by decomposing bleaching powder with dry sodium carbonate in the proportion of 150 gm. to 105 gm., dissolved in one liter of water. The mixture is filtered and a measured portion of it (20 c.c.) rapidly titrated with a boric acid solution of known strength (31 gm. per liter, ½ normal), using phenolphthalein suspended in water as indicator (the usual alcoholic solution of phenolphthalein will not serve, because the alcohol is at once attacked) in order to determine the amount of boric acid to be added to the rest of the filtrate. (Each cubic centimeter of N/2 boric acid calls for 3 gm. boric acid to be added.) An excess of boric acid should be avoided, as it favors the liberation of hypochlorous acid and renders the solution less stable. It is best to add slightly less than the calculated amount. The concentrated solution thus prepared contains about 4 per cent. of sodium hypochlorite and should be mixed with 7 parts of water before use. It can be kept for a month without serious decomposition.

Titration of Bleaching Powder.—The variation in the strength of the commercial products makes it necessary to determine the amount of active chlorin in the bleaching powder. Exactly 10 gm. of bleaching powder, made up of small samples from different parts of the jar, in order to obtain a representative sample, are well stirred up in a liter of water. After standing about six hours the solution is filtered and a 10 c.c. sample of the filtrate is titrated in exactly the same manner as in the titration of Dakin's solution. In this case the number of cubic centimeters of decinormal thiosulphate required to decolorize, multiplied by the factor 3.55, gives the percentage of active chlorin in the bleaching powder.

"Dakin's hypochlorite solutions possess the property of dissolving necrotic tissue, and therefore should be used as long as there is any such tissue to be dissolved. Whenever the wound is cleaned up and only mildly infected, it is desirable to substitute the chloramin paste. This paste has no solvent action at all on necrotic tissue, but is an efficient antiseptic. It is applied about once a day." The formula follows:

Preparation of Daufresne Chloramin-T Paste.*—Prepare, in hot water, a 7.5 per cent. solution of sodium stearate, either from the pure salt or by neutralizing 696 gm. of stearic acid with 98 gm. of sodium hydroxid to make 10 liters of paste. Neutral-

* Daufresne, Jour. Exper. Med., xxvi, 91, 1917.

ize the free alkali in this solution by adding a concentrated boric acid solution until a slight cloudiness (due to precipitated stearic acid) appears, or until 5 c.c. mixed with 5 c.c. 95 per cent. alcohol gives no color to phenolphthalein. Then pour the hot solution into a mixing machine (an ordinary ice-cream freezer, for example), the container of which is surrounded by hot water. The container should not be more than three-quarters full. A hole should be bored at the bottom of the wooden bucket for the introduction of cold water, which should be allowed gradually to reduce the temperature. Begin introducing the cold water as soon as the machine starts, and so regulate the flow that the complete cooling will take about one and a quarter hours. Then open the container, and if the paste looks smooth and has no granulations, add enough chloramin-T (also known commercially as *"chlorazene"*) dissolved in a little water to make a 1 per cent. paste. Again allow the machine to beat the paste for thirty minutes. The paddles of the mixer must turn very slowly—about 30 revolutions per minute. The paste may be kept for several weeks.

Titration of the chloramin-T content: Place 10 gm. of the paste in an Erlenmeyer flask with water and titrate with iodid and acid, exactly as for Dakin's solution. The precipitated stearic acid does not interfere. Multiply the number of cubic centimeters of thiosulphate solution required to decolorize by 0.141 to obtain the percentage of chloramin-T.

THE CARREL-DAKIN METHOD

Technic of the Dressing.
—"*Necessary Materials.*—
1. An antiseptic: Dakin's hypochlorite solution, or chloramin-T (also known as chlorazene) or chloramin-T paste.

"2. A glass container with a capacity of from 500 to 1000 c.c. (Fig. 24, *a*).

"3. Two yards of moderate-sized rubber tubing.

"4. An adjustable clamp for controlling the flow of the solution (Fig. 24, *c*).

"5. Rubber instillation tubes about 25 cm. long, with assorted diameters (average size, 4 mm. inside diameter). These tubes are tied at the extremity and perforated with holes made with a punch. The primary and secondary tubes are 7 mm. in internal diameter, the final distributing tubes 4 mm., and the little holes in these tubes are only 1 mm. ($\frac{1}{25}$ inch) in diameter.

"6. Similar tubes which

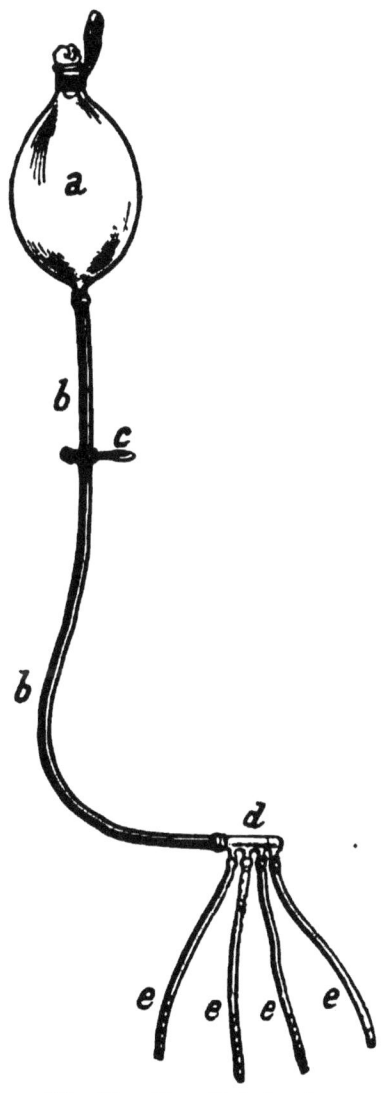

Fig. 24.—Carrel's irrigation apparatus: *a*, Reservoir for Dakin's fluid; *b, b*, the main distributing tube; *c*, the metal pinch-cock; *d*, glass tube with multiple openings; *e, e, e, e*, final distributing tubes closed at distal end, but perforated with openings of 1 mm. each (Carrel and Dehelly).

are not ligated, and which have a small lateral opening near one end.

"7. Glass connecting and distributing tubes (Fig. 27).

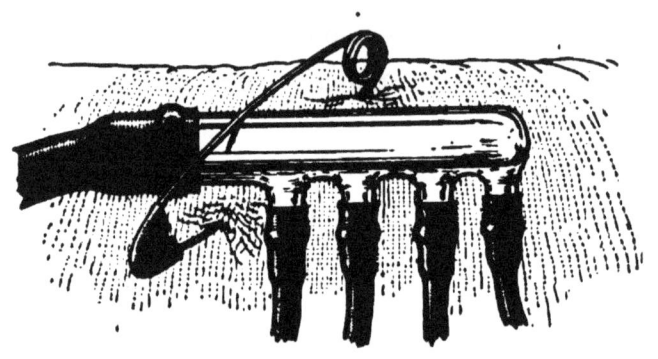

Fig. 25.—Showing Carrel's glass tube (Fig. 24, *d*) to connect the main distributing tube (Fig. 24, *b, b*) from the reservoir to multiple final small distributing tubes (Carrel and Dehelly).

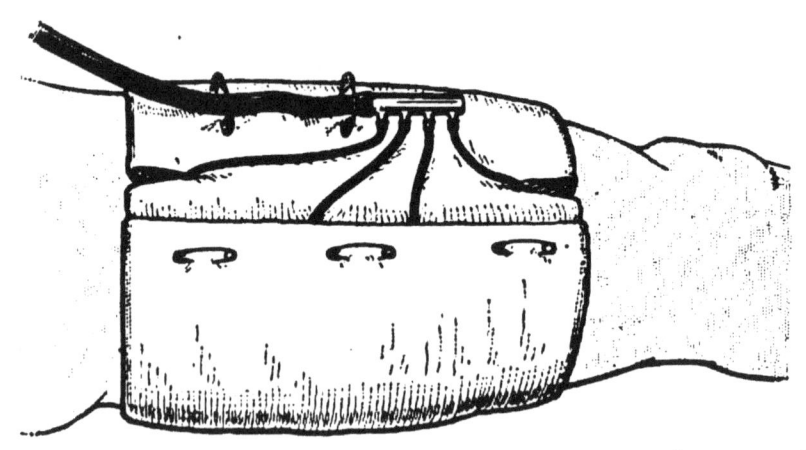

Fig. 26.—Showing the mode in which the small distributing tubes are carried through the dressing to the various parts of the wound (Carrel and Dehelly).

"8. The *dressings* consist of cotton surrounded by gauze. The cotton consists of a layer of absorbent cotton with a thicker layer of non-absorbent cotton.

These dressings are about 3 cm. thick, and of different sizes. Three different sizes are sufficient—one large enough to surround the leg once, a second to surround the arm, the third still smaller. Safety-pins on bandages fasten the dressing in place.

"9. Sterilized pieces of gauze impregnated with yellow petrolatum to be used in the protection of the skin.

"**Operative Technic to Prepare the Wound for the Introduction of the Antiseptic.**—The future course of the wound is directly dependent on the thoroughness

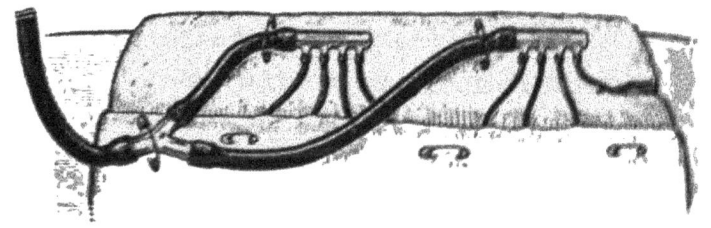

Fig. 27.—Showing a similar distribution as in Fig. 26, by means of a Y-tube, thus doubling the number of final distributing tubes (Carrel and Dehelly).

of the first surgical act. This should be carried out under the strictest aseptic precaution and at the earliest possible moment. It consists of a thorough, methodical, mechanical disinfection of the wound, with the extraction of all shell fragments, particles of clothing, dirt, etc. [For the methods of locating and extracting foreign bodies see p. 123.]

"The operative field is painted with tincture of iodin, and the bruised and necrotic skin-edges of the wound are trimmed away with a sharp knife. The knife and forceps are then put aside. With new instru-

98 TREATMENT OF WAR WOUNDS

ments the wound is laid open like a book and gently explored for shell fragments, pieces of clothing, pockets, etc. Everything that could have been infected by the traumatism or could become the source of infection is removed. All non-infected tissues and tissues unlikely to become infected are preserved.

"Gentleness of manipulation is the keystone of the technic. Brutalization of the traumatized tissue is a technical crime. In many of the cases it will be found that fibers of clothing, dirt, grass, etc., are encrusted in the muscular sur-

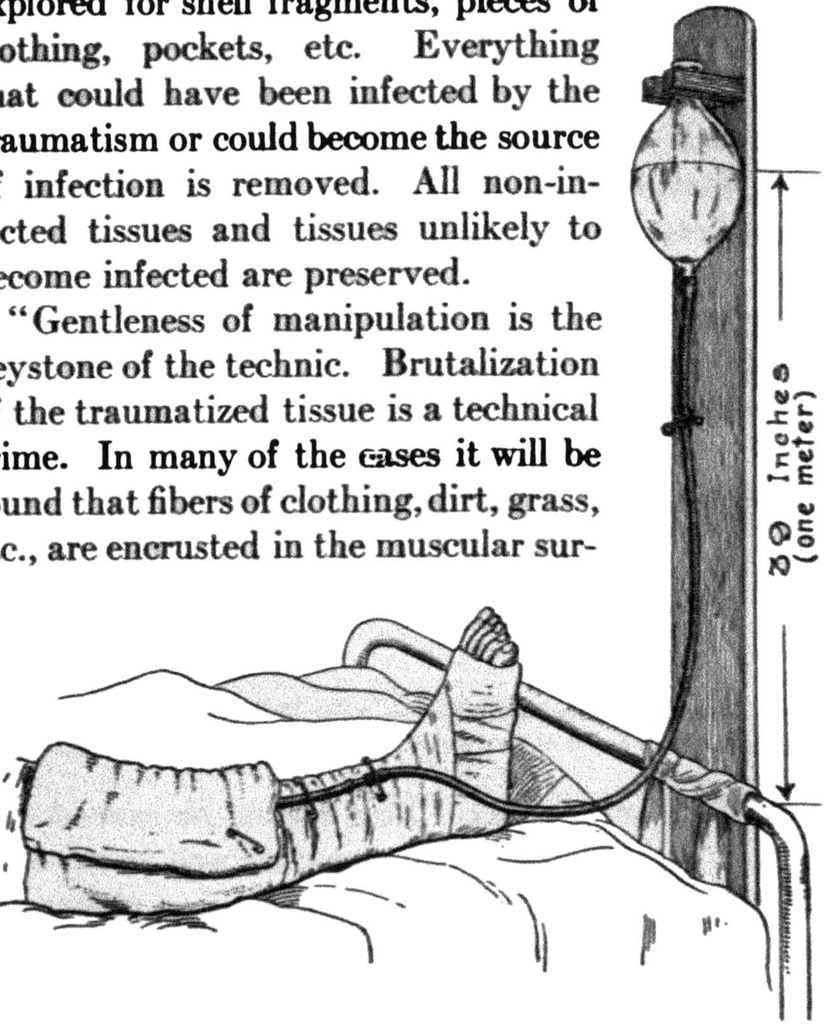

Fig. 28.—Showing Carrel method of irrigating wound with the Dakin fluid. Note on the main distributing tube the pinch-cock below the reservoir. The wound is covered with the dressing, which is fastened by safety-pins. The distributing tube is similarly held in place by being pinned outside of the dressing (Carrel and Dehelly modified).

faces of the wounds. To avoid overlooking this blood-débris the track of the projectile must be lightly but methodically resected. Great conservatism is exercised in the removal of comminuted fragments of bone. The same minute and careful mechanical cleansing is carried out in osseous wounds as in the soft parts. Before placing the instillation tubes, a careful revision of the wound is made, and particular attention paid to securing a perfect hemostasis.

"Vessels are ligated (plain catgut being used). Oozing is stopped by pressure or by a hot saline solution. This hemostasis is thoroughly made for two reasons: Because bacteria may remain located in blood-clots which are dissolved by Dakin's solution very slowly and because blood may plug the tubes.

"In cases of *suppurating wounds*, the infection is reduced as much as possible by chemical means, the necessary surgical cleansing is then performed, and is followed by a new and thorough chemical treatment.

"Counter-openings for drainage are rarely employed. If the necessity for their use should arise, one should avoid making them at the most dependent point, as the goal of technic is to keep the liquid in contact with *all* the surfaces of the wound.

"**The Introduction of the Instillation Tubes.**—The guiding principle is to place the tubes so that the liquid will come into contact with every portion of the wound, taking into consideration the principle of gravity. The placing of the tubes will vary with the nature of the wound.

The skin surrounding the wound is then coated with yellow vaselin (not white) to prevent irritation.

"*Superficial Wounds.*—The requisite number of tubes are inserted first directly in contact with the wound. They are affixed to the surface of the surrounding skin by means of strips of adhesive plaster, in order to prevent their disturbance. The arrangement of the tubes in the wound is maintained by compresses of gauze loosely packed.

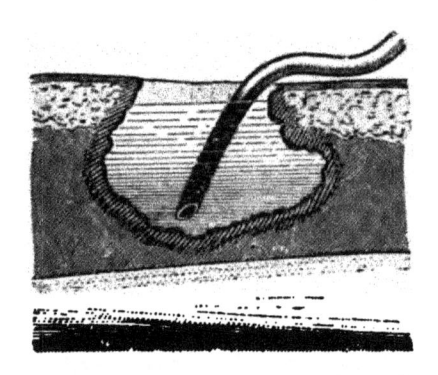

Fig. 29.—Showing Carrel's method of using Dakin's solution in an anterior wound and keeping the wound full of the solution like a cup, so as constantly to attack the infecting bacteria (Carrel and Dehelly).

"*Penetrating Wounds.*— In the simple type, a tube without lateral perforations is introduced to the depth of the cavity and the solution allowed to well up from the bottom (Fig. 29). In a large tract terminating in a cavity with irregular collapsible walls a little gauze is introduced to support the walls of the cavity and allow a more thorough distribution of the fluid, tubes being inserted first close to the walls. Penetrating wounds with the point of entrance in a dependent position (as the buttock, posterior surface of the extremities, and the back) are treated with perforated tubes dressed with toweling (Fig. 31). These dressed tubes keep the antiseptic in contact with the wound. A tube with a single hole can also be used.

THE CARREL-DAKIN METHOD

"*Through-and-through Wounds.*—A perforated tube with the tied extremity uppermost is passed from the lower to the upper wound. The liquid, escaping through the small lateral holes, flows back along the

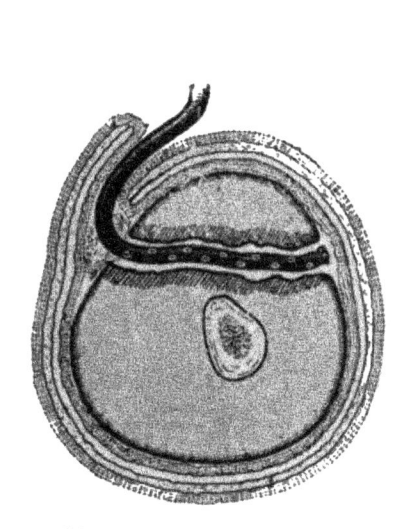

Fig. 30.—Showing the method by which the distributing tube enters the wound through the dressing without being constricted (Carrel and Dehelly).

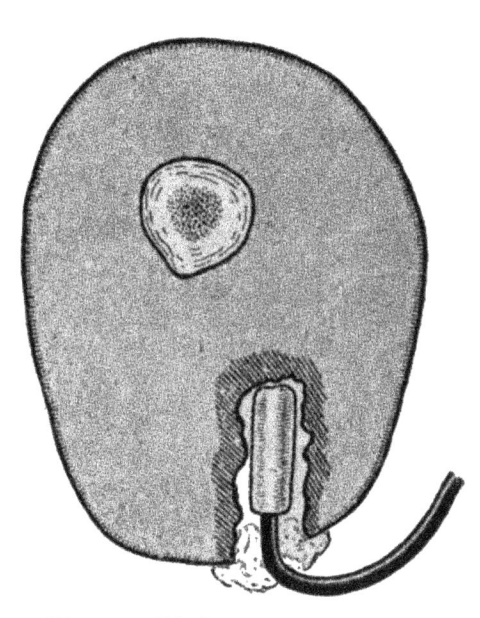

Fig. 31.—Mode of irrigating a wound in a posterior position. Observe that the distributing tube is here necessarily surrounded with toweling, otherwise the fluid would escape almost immediately. This toweling should be firmly sewed to the distributing tube (*b*, Fig. 24, p. 95) by silk and not by catgut, so that it may not become detached and be left in the wound (Carrel and Dehelly).

tract to the inferior orifice, moistening the entire wound.

"Wounds of the hand or foot, open amputation stumps, etc., are immersed in Dakin's solution for

102   TREATMENT OF WAR WOUNDS

from ten to fifteen minutes every two hours until the wound is sterilized. The skin is protected by smearing it with sterile yellow petrolatum.

"**The After-care of the Wounds.**—The materials used are described above. In the care of the wounds

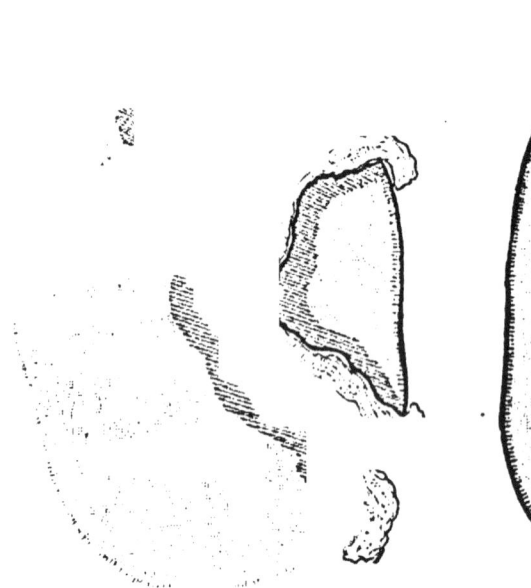

Fig. 32.—Showing the *improper* way of placing the distributing tubes. They are in contact with the gauze instead of in contact with the wound (Carrel and Dehelly).

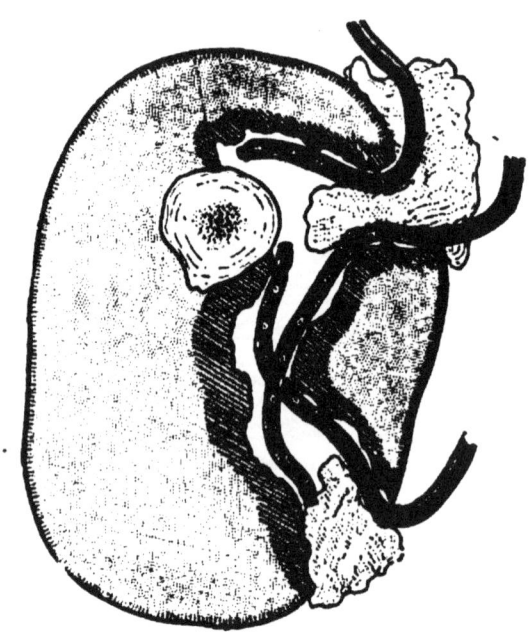

Fig. 33.—The *correct* way of placing the distributing tubes so that the Dakin fluid comes directly in contact with all the surfaces of the wound (Carrel and Dehelly).

a strict instrumental technic is employed, even the gloved hands never coming in contact with the wounds or dressings.

"Instillations of the fluid are made every two hours [day and night] by releasing the adjustable clamp [for a second or two] (Fig. 27) controlling the flow. The amount of solution employed varies with the nature and extent of the wound; for the average wound, 40 c.c. are sufficient. This interrupted instillation is kept up until the wound is proved sterile. The tubes are then removed, and a compress moistened with Dakin's solution is applied. Formerly a continuous instillation was the method of choice. The rate of instillation is from 5 to 20 drops a minute, according to conditions. The object is to moisten the wound surfaces with fresh solution.

"Once a day the dressing is applied, and the wound, the tubes, and the flow of the liquid are inspected. Flushing the wound shows if the solution is being delivered as planned. Secretions are removed with a cotton sponge slightly moistened with sterile water.

"The Carrel method is not a continuous irrigation. It is a mechanical attempt to deliver an antiseptic of definite chemical concentration to every portion of a surgically prepared wound and to insure its constant contact for a prolonged period. (*Cf.* pp. 95 *et seqq.*)

"Systematic Bacteriologic Examination of the Wound.—This consists in a regular determination of the number of microbes on the wound surfaces. This is done by transferring with a standard loop a portion of the secretion to a slide and counting the number of microbes per microscopic field. This is carried out every second day, and the results are entered on a suitable chart. When the bacteria are so reduced in number that only one is found per five or ten microscopic fields, the wound is considered as 'surgically' sterile. The bacteriologic control is indispensable. Clinical examination is impotent to give the necessary information.

"The bacterial chart is begun the first time the wound is examined. By it the different stages of the disinfection are followed. As the wounded arrive usually not earlier than ten or twelve hours after injury, the number of bacteria is relatively small because they are diluted with blood. Twenty-four hours after the injury their number is infinite. There is an initial rise on the second or third day. This remains so for a few days, and then the descent begins. Wounds of the soft parts are sterilized in from five to eight days. Greatly traumatized wounds require a longer time. Fractures can be sterilized in from two to four weeks. If sequestra are present, they must be removed to obtain an asepsis.

"Wounds sterilized by the Carrel method are readily reinfected if the treatment is stopped.

"Reunion of Wound.—When, by three successive tests, the bacteriologic examination shows the wound to be sterile, it is closed. In the favorable cases this can be done on the fifth day. The average time for the soft parts is from seven to nine days.

"The wounds are closed by adhesive straps passed in such a way that, besides pulling the edges of the wound together, they make a compression around the whole circumference of the limb, or a 'corset lacing'

(Fig. 34). Care must be taken not to have the circular bandage, if this be used, too tight.

"For extensive wounds two Canton-flannel bands are prepared, the length to be slightly longer than the wound, the breadth to be a little less than half the circumference of the limb. On the hemmed edges shoe-hooks are inserted every 2 cm. The limbs are painted up to the edges of the wound with a resin varnish or Heusner's glue (see page 52), and the woolly side of the Canton flannel applied. One

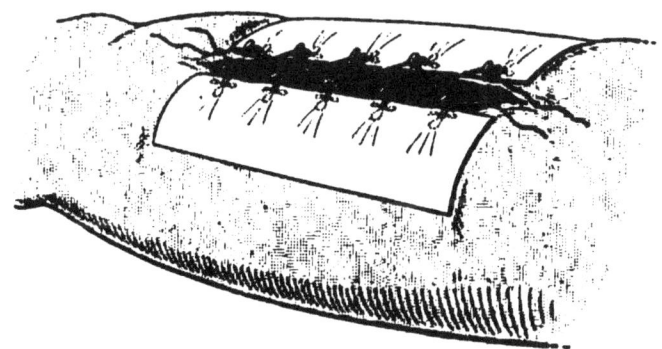

Fig. 34.—The edges of a wound being drawn together by rubber elastic traction (Carrel and Dehelly).

should wait until the traction strips are firmly adherent before lacing them with rubber bands. The tension of the rubber bands rapidly draws the wound edges together. When, after the twelfth day, the skin is adherent to the deeper structures and not movable, closure of the wound must be made by suture after excision of the epithelial edge."

In the entire treatment of these wounds even the gloved hands never are allowed to touch any dressing or the wound. Everything is handled by forceps, which can be so much more certainly disinfected than hands or even gloves.

When a wound has filled up and is in condition to cicatrize, Carrel and Lecompte du Noüy, a French

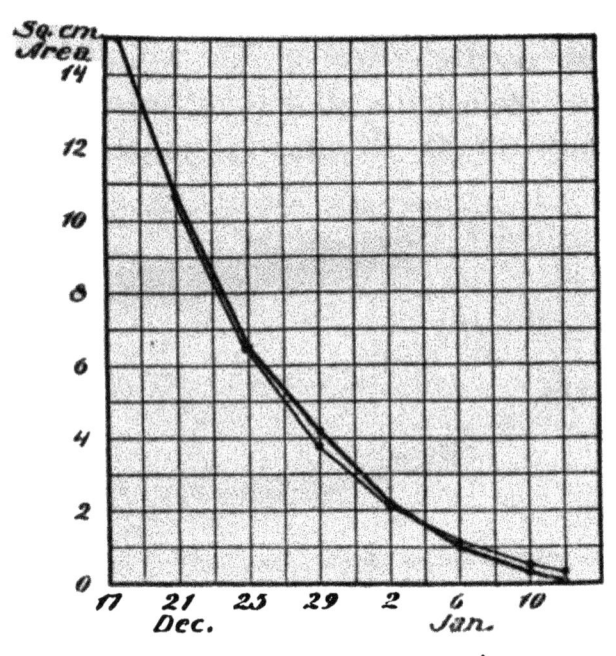

Fig. 35.—On December 17th the area of the wound was 16.2 sq. cm. A slight infection between December 27th and 29th, when one microörganism in two microscopic fields was found, caused a slight deviation of the actual curve from the calculated curve. (Kindness of Carrel and du Noüy and the Jour. Exp. Med., 1916, xxiv, 454.)

physicist, by means of a "planimeter," are able to measure the exact area, *i. e.*, the number of square centimeters, of a superficial wound no matter how irregular the outline. The number of square centimeters is entered on a chart (Figs. 35, 36, 37, vertical numbers) every second day. The dates are entered

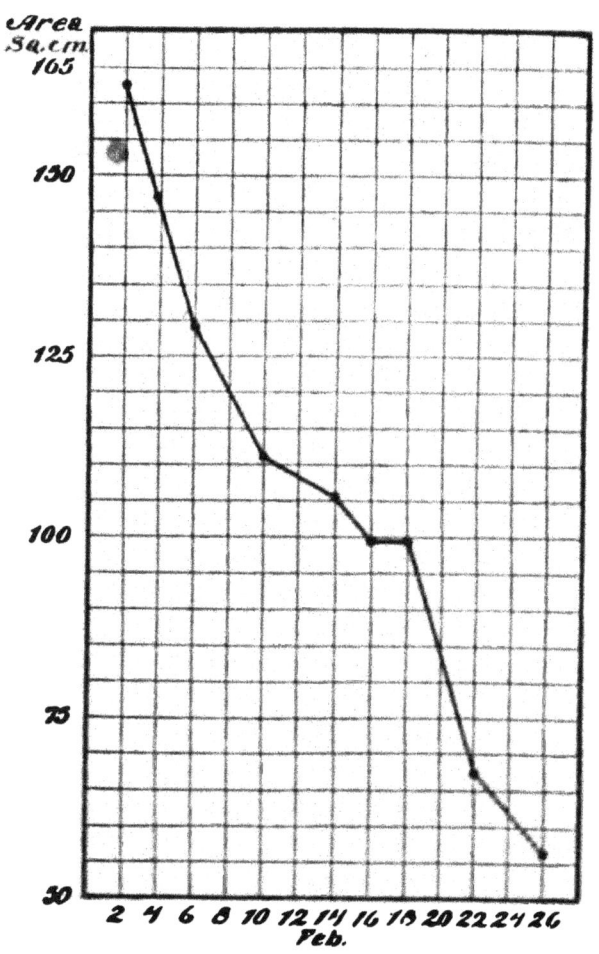

Fig. 36.—Wound of the abdominal wall. The horizontal part of the curve from February 16th to 18th represents a period of slight infection. As soon as the wound was sterilized chemically the curve descended abruptly. (Kindness of Carrel and Hartman and the Jour. Exp. Med., 1916, xxiv, p. 457.)

below the chart (the horizontal numbers). After three or four observations have been entered, a "curve of healing" is established. By prolonging this curve they can predict with accuracy the day on which a given superficial wound will be completely healed.

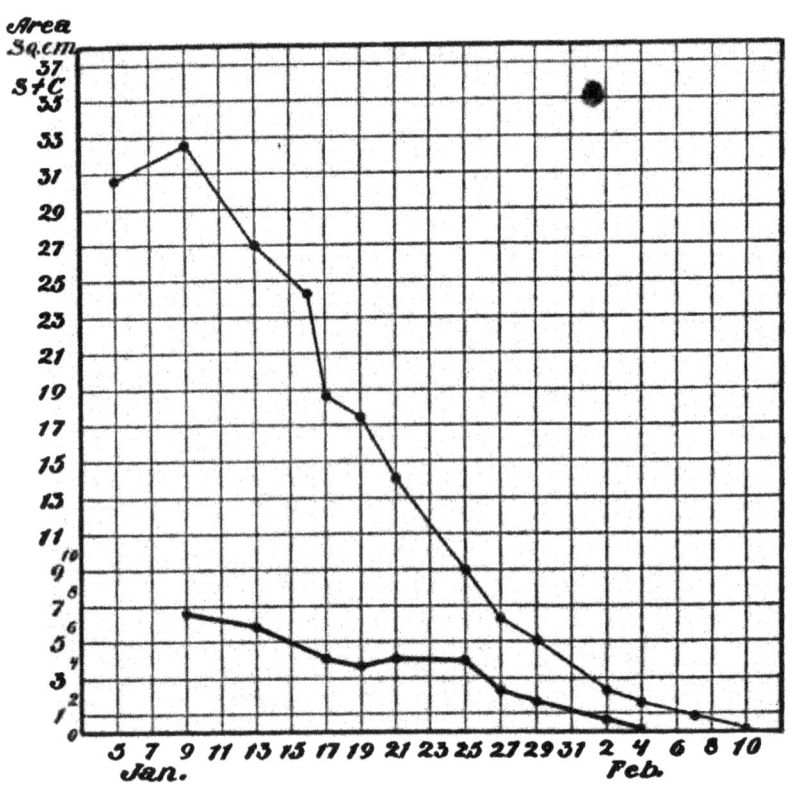

Fig. 37.—Shell wounds with fracture of the radius and ulna. The curves of both wounds tend to unite. Note that the larger wound, 33 sq. cm., healed far more rapidly than the smaller wound, which was less than 7 sq. cm. on the same date. (Kindness of Carrel and Hartman and the Jour. Exp. Med., 1916, xxiv, p. 442.)

It is remarkable how nearly the "actual" curve and the "calculated" curve in a normal case coincide (Fig. 35). Any renewed infection, of course, disturbs the observed curve, but, curiously enough, if the infection is quickly overcome, the healing process undergoes acceleration and the healing will still be brought about at or very near the predicted date. Of course, any prolonged infection would considerably delay the healing. Another curious fact brought out by these curves is that large wounds heal much more rapidly than small wounds (Fig. 37). (The whole subject is treated at length in the Journal of Experimental Medicine, 1916, vol. xxiv, pp. 451–470.)

In spite of its immense value, four valid objections to the Carrel-Dakin method are evident:

1. The irritation of the skin, an irritation which sometimes is very painful and may persist for a long time. To minimize this it is essential not only to protect the skin by yellow vaselin, but that minute care also be taken to insure the exact strength of the solution. Below 0.40 per cent. the germicidal action is too feeble. Above 0.50 per cent. the solution is too irritating. This means that the solution must be most carefully made and tested and that fresh solutions must be constantly prepared (*cf.* p. 88).

2. The solutions, when in contact with the wound exudates, lose their chlorin in an hour or even less time and become inert. Hence the need of a new supply of the fluid every two hours. This constant care,

day and night, the care not to use too much or too little, the expense of so much solution, apparatus, and dressing, etc., make the method time-consuming and costly. Above all, it requires a large staff of doctors and nurses.

3. In order to obtain the maximum germicidal effect of weak hypochlorite solutions it is necessary to keep them in *constant* contact with all surfaces of the wound. In the Carrel-Dakin technic this is accomplished by making basin-like cavities of all the wounds. This means that dependent—*i. e.*, the most efficient—drainage must be avoided.

4. It is impossible to keep up the treatment during transit for any distance. The chloramin-T paste (p. 93), while much less desirable at this stage, can be substituted, as it usually requires only one daily dressing.

In spite of these difficulties Depage, at LaPanne, in a large hospital, is most successfully using the Carrel-Dakin treatment. They are not, therefore, insuperable.

DICHLORAMIN-T

This is a new chlorin compound introduced by Dakin and described in Dakin and Dunham's Handbook of Antiseptics (ed. 1918, pp. 33 *et seqq.*). It contains twice as much chlorin as the chloramin-T, and has a much stronger germicidal action. It can also be used up to a strength of 5 per cent., 10 per cent., and even 20 per cent. For general surgical purposes a 5 per cent. to an 8 per cent. solution is strong enough.

It is but slightly soluble in water. At first it was dissolved in chlorinated eucalyptol and paraffin oil. Dakin's present method of preparing dichloramin-T and its solutions are as follows:*

In oily solutions usually "intimate contact with the infected matter is hindered by the oil," and hence the solutions possess little antiseptic activity. In this preparation, however, a certain amount of the dichloramin-T passes into the watery warmed fluids and so exerts its germicidal action. "The oil solution serves as a store of the antiseptic which is drawn

* Dakin and Dunham's Handbook of Antiseptics, Ed. 1918, pp. 37–40.

upon to maintain the germicidal activity" in the wound fluids.

It is most conveniently applied by means of an oil spray (Fig. 38). If the solution is too thick, add

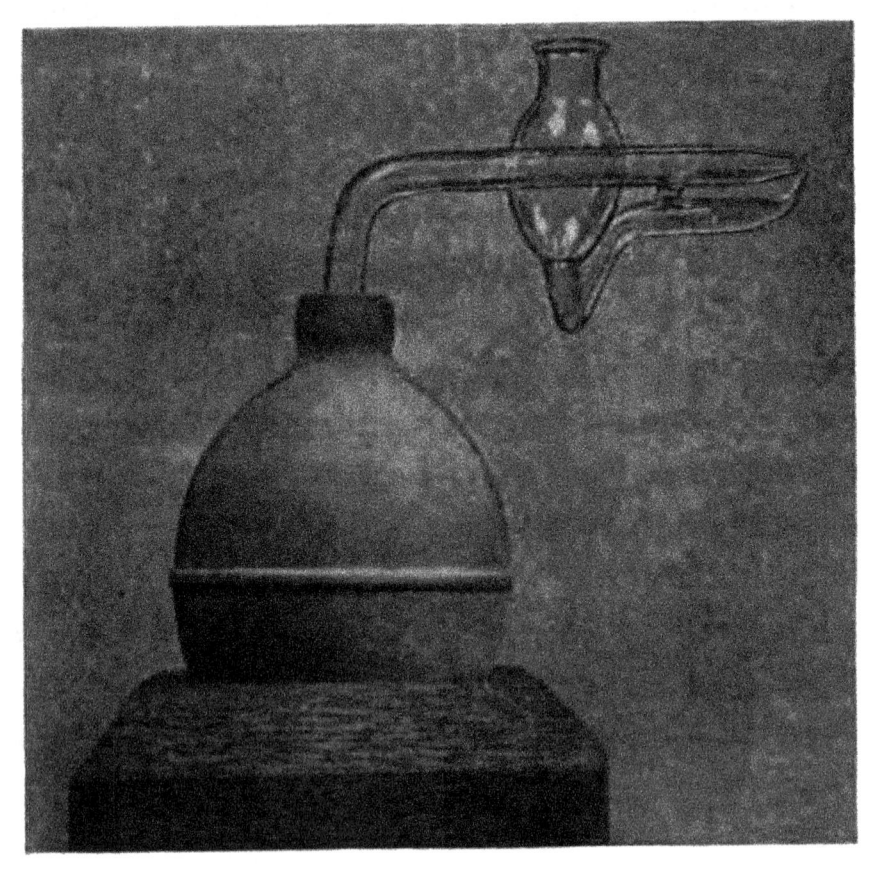

Fig. 38.—Apparatus for spraying the dichloramin-T solution on wounds (courtesy of Capt. W. Estell Lee).

10 per cent. in volume of carbon tetrachlorid. This is added only just when the oil is to be sprayed. The undiluted solution can be used in a wound even in

the abdomen (*vide* p. 116), or it can be introduced into a cavity by a glass syringe (Fig. 39). One or 2 c.c. are enough for an ordinary wound. Only enough for the wounds to be treated should be poured out for immediate use. The unused portion should be thrown away and not returned to the stock bottle.

All stock solutions "must be kept in *amber glass* bottles since direct sunlight causes rapid decomposition. *Blue glass affords no protection.*"

The germicidal action of dichloramin-T continues for eighteen to twenty-four hours. In solution it is said not to affect the body cells, even in the stronger percentages. The dressing, therefore, is done only once a day; the technic is simple and permits dependent drainage. There is a great saving of material, and, what is of greater consequence, the time given to each case, except

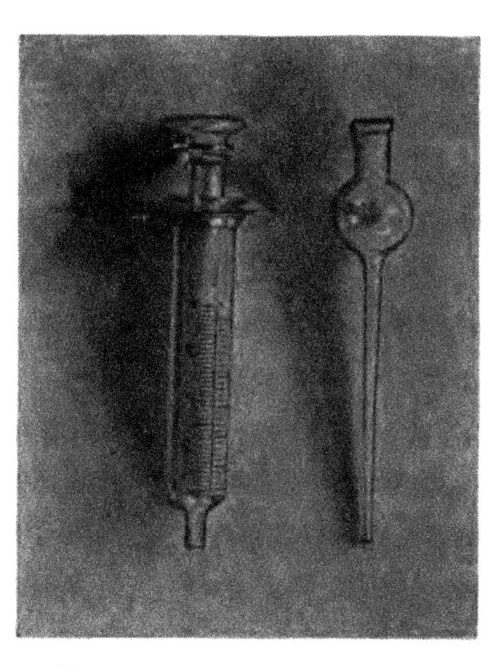

Fig. 39.—Syringe for injecting the dichloramin-T solution into wound cavities (courtesy of Capt. W. Estell Lee).

at the primary operation or dressing, is greatly reduced.

The Technic.*—The most rigid aseptic ritual is observed. Gowns, gloves on sterilized hands, neither the wound nor any dressing is ever touched even by the gloved hand. Everything is handled by sterile forceps. The moment these instruments are even possibly soiled they are discarded for freshly sterilized ones. As it cannot be sterilized, the atomizer for spraying on the oil is manipulated by a nurse.

The skin is cleansed by soap and water, but is carefully dried and then washed with benzene. This cannot be used more than once or twice. Neither alcohol nor peroxid of hydrogen should be used, as they decompose the dichloramin-T. The skin-wound and all the devitalized tissue in the track of the wound which can properly be excised anatomically are removed, in one piece if possible. If practicable, the entire wound is laid open to facilitate this removal. All foreign bodies, especially clothing, are removed.

Every bleeding vessel must be tied. The fresh surface is then well sprayed over with the dichloramin-T solution and immediately sutured, always without

---

* Abstracted from Captains Lee and Furness, "Treatment of Infections and Infected Wounds with Dichloramin-T." This paper will be soon published in the *Military Surgeon*.

drainage. As the dichloramin-T does not affect the tensile strength nor the holding of catgut knots, secondary hemorrhage is eliminated. Sweet reports from France that there was not a single case among 1200 infected major wounds. Only a light dressing of three or four layers of gauze is used. This effected at the Pennsylvania Hospital a saving of 75 per cent. of gauze—an important economic item. The saving of time for the surgeon and his assistants, especially if they are well trained to work as a "team," is even more important and more time- and money-saving.

In case infection occurs, one or two stitches are cut and the oil is introduced by the glass syringe (Fig. 39).

In all redressings the outer non-sterile bandages or dressings are removed by the patient himself if he is able, or by a nurse if he is not; the dressing next the wound is removed by the surgeon himself with sterile forceps, which are immediately replaced by freshly sterilized forceps.

In older infected wounds, after laying the wound open and removing all devitalized tissues and foreign bodies if present, adequate drainage should be provided. The wound-edges are held apart by a generous gauze pack saturated with the oil and a four-ply outer dressing applied.

Light gauze bandages or adhesive plaster is used to retain the dressings in place.

In intra-abdominal wounds and operations naturally Lee and Furness began with great caution to apply the oil in old, well-walled-off sinuses following operations for appendicitis and tubal abscesses. Emboldened by their good results they are now using the method in such walled-off cavities at the time of operation. After removal of a gangrenous or perforated appendix "the 5 per cent. solution is dropped over all the visibly affected tissue. A medium-sized gauze drain (Mikulicz) saturated with the same strength of oil is then packed into the cavity and the wound partially closed. . . . The later dressings consist in applying 2 or 3 c.c. of the oil . . . to the gauze wick and the edges of the wound. After forty-eight hours the gauze wick is easily removed." As soon as the drain is loosened (three to seven days) it is removed.

The clinical results, both in civil and in military practice, seem to promise well.

At the Pennsylvania Hospital in Philadelphia, Dakin, Lee, Sweet, Hendrix, and LeConte (Jour. Amer. Med. Assoc., July 7, 1917) have made comparative clinical tests, with the following results:

In 160 unselected cases of industrial accidents

treated by the Carrel-Dakin method the Carrel-Dakin cases were discharged in one-third of the time required by former methods (as obtained from the industrial insurance statistics of similar cases in other Philadelphia hospitals)—a great advantage.

In 82 similar unselected cases treated in the same clinic by the Dichloramin-T-in-oil method they were discharged in 16.3 per cent. less time than by the Carrel-Dakin method—a still better result. These results, however, were obtained under the favorable conditions of civil life, in a first-class hospital, and in the absence of the intense infection seen in the present war.

THE "BIPP" TREATMENT OF MR. RUTHERFORD MORISON, OF NEWCASTLE-ON-TYNE*

The name is derived from the initial letters of *bismuth* (one ounce by weight), *iodoform* (two ounces by weight), liquid *paraffin*, sufficient (usually about one ounce) to make a thick *paste*, which indicate its composition and physical character. Rub it down in small quantities with a spatula on a slab to eliminate any grit. Morison's claim is that "by a few dressings many wounds can be sterilized at once [*i. e.*, immediately.—K.], while in the remainder," so far as his experience goes, "the spread of infection can be checked and remedied."

The general surgical principle underlying the whole method is thus stated: "If it be possible to get to the bottom of an infected wound, so that it can be thoroughly cleansed mechanically and suitable antiseptics be applied, the wound can then be closed with interrupted sutures, always with impunity, and many times with the prospect of seeing it healed when the

*See his papers in the Lancet, August 12, 1916, Brit. Jour. Surg., April, 1917, Brit. Med. Jour., October 20, 1917, and International Jour. Surg., February, 1918.

dressing is removed for the first time at the end of three weeks. This is a new surgical principle which will not alter, though details of the method will."

His directions for its use are briefly as follows:

1. Clean the skin and surrounding area by carbolic solution 1 : 20, usually under an anesthetic.

2. Open the wound freely, down to the bottom if possible, preserving especially nerves and their muscular branches. Cleanse the cavity with dry sterile mops, Volkmann's spoon, etc., and remove all foreign bodies.

3. Mop the surrounding skin and the wound cavity with methylated spirit (wood alcohol) and dry it.

4. Fill the whole cavity with hipp, rubbing it well in with dry gauze. *Remove all excess*, leaving only a thin covering over the wounded surface. [Cases of bismuth or iodoform *poisoning* have been reported from *neglect* of this important direction.—K.] Dress the wound with sterile gauze and an absorbent pad held in place by adhesive plaster and a bandage.

If the patient is free from pain and constitutional disturbance, this primary dressing may be left in place for days or even weeks. "If discharge comes through, the stained part must be soaked in the spirit and a gauze dressing wrung out of the same applied as a further covering."

"Redressing is very simply done. After removal of the old dressing the wound is covered with a dossil of wool soaked in spirit, and the sticky, dirty-looking discharge is wiped off the surrounding skin until it is clean."

In gunshot fractures "after reduction of the fracture they are splinted and left without redressing for from two to six weeks, so that, after the operation, they are no more trouble than are simple fractures," either to the patient or the surgeon. "The end results in a considerable proportion are not even yet sufficiently good to satisfy the most moderate surgical ambition, and there is room for great improvement." Early in the war the results of plating were so bad that it was forbidden by the War Office. Now, and especially under the bipp treatment, Morison believes that plating may safely be done—but only "by surgeons who have had exceptional experience and who have a hospital team under their control."

Necrosis, as it is the result of infection, does not occur in the majority of recent fractures treated by bipp. This means an enormous conservation of man power.

Suppurating sinuses leading to similar bone cavities, after thorough disinfection by bipp, can be filled with fatty tissue and will heal.

Five cases of wound of the knee-joint then in his ward treated with bipp in France arrived without pain or constitutional disturbance and with "already fair movement of the joint."

In cerebral hernia its use has been very satisfactory, the dressing being left for more than a week. The hernia healed in twelve to twenty-four days.

In amputations it has been equally satisfactory. The dressings should remain unchanged for three weeks. The sutures may then be removed—not earlier, lest the wound reopen in parts.

The objections are—First, the danger of gas gangrene after such closure of the wound by sutures. This danger he thinks can be avoided by packing the wound with sulphate of magnesia cream or with gauze wrung out of flavine solution for, say, four days, after which he thinks there is no probability of an outbreak. [As Mr. Morison's experience, I understand, is wholly in England, this statement would have to be checked up by surgeons at the front itself.—K.]

A second objection is that the paste, being impervious to the x-ray, hinders all x-ray pictures. This can be avoided by the same means as the first objection. During these three or four days x-ray pictures can be freely taken.

A third objection has already been mentioned—the danger of bismuth or iodoform poisoning and the importance of rubbing off all excess of the paste. If this is done with care, there seems to be little chance of harm. (*Cf.* Bowlby's letter, p. 244.)

LOCALIZATION AND REMOVAL OF FOREIGN BODIES BY X-RAYS

LOCALIZATION OF FOREIGN BODIES

There is perhaps no phase of war surgery in which x-ray examination may play so helpful a rôle as in determining the presence of dense foreign bodies, and in ascertaining with a suitable degree of accuracy their anatomic position.

At the beginning of the present war the methods in general use were essentially those developed several years ago. These usually involved considerable mechanical apparatus, and also the development and later mensuration of shadows on photographic negatives. There had been developed for surgical localization of small foreign bodies in the eye a very satisfactory and simple apparatus which seems not to have been improved upon in recent years. In a book of moderate size, like the present one, it is evidently necessary to select from the great variety of methods only those that seem to satisfy certain essential conditions.

A satisfactory method of localization for military hospitals, where speed and simplicity are essential, must, of necessity, be independent of the use of photography, as time will not permit, and the facilities may often be inadequate for the proper handling of plates or films. When we review also the conditions under which this work must be done, and the necessity for avoiding all methods which are especially liable to introduce errors, only methods of the greatest degree of simplicity, both as to apparatus and the necessary measurements or computations, can be described.

It is also very desirable that such simple apparatus be adopted as will eliminate computations and relieve the roentgenologist from giving attention to minor details, in order that he may devote himself more specifically to the anatomic localization.

After a careful consideration of the methods already in use, it has been decided to confine the work of instruction and the apparatus supplied to six fairly well-known methods, with such modifications as would tend to insure the greatest accuracy and rapidity in the work.

In this connection it should be remarked that geometric or academic accuracy, which must always be the ideal of the roentgenologist, with the single exception of a few cases, as the eye or head, is not absolutely essential to the surgeon. This fact cannot excuse, however, any lack of painstaking accuracy.

The chief of our x-Ray Division in France has said, "This war is not being fought with bird shot." Geometric measurement, however accurate, must be translated by the surgeon into the invisible regions within the patient's body, and it must be remembered that the position of a foreign body is modified at once when incisions are made and retractors used in the course of operation. For this reason an effort is being made to train roentgenologists not simply to say that the projectile is at a certain depth within the tissue below a certain skin-mark, but to give much more important data as to its location with reference to surgical and anatomic landmarks.

We may divide localization methods into two distinct groups, one of which gives a depth measurement in the so-called vertical direction, below a skin-mark, and *which assumes that the patient will be placed in the same position for operation as he was during the x-ray examination, and that the surgeon looks exactly in the direction taken by the ray during examination by the roentgenologist.* Needless to say that in many cases these conditions cannot be realized and there may be a consequent failure to utilize properly the information given to the surgeon. In other cases, in addition to an indication of depth, there is given some sort of a surgical guide to aid the surgeon before or during operation.

It just happens that of the methods selected by the x-Ray Division of the army there are three of each type, and it is left for the roentgenologist, in coöperation with the surgeon, to decide in what cases something more than a mere statement of depth from a skin-mark is necessary. It should also be remembered that in base hospitals more time can be allowed and more extensive equipment may be provided than would reasonably be expected nearer the front.

In the description and instruction sheets it has been deemed wise to omit the names of those generally regarded as responsible for the introduction of particular methods, partly because the literature available is rarely accurate as regards priority, but more important still, because the roentgenologist is liable to find in the literature instructions quite at variance with those given for the use of our standard apparatus, which may result in confusion and inaccuracy. The methods are therefore designated as A, B, C, D, E, and F, of which the first three are without surgical indicators and the last three have some indicator in addition to ordinary depth localization. Furthermore, these are arranged in the

LOCALIZATION OF FOREIGN BODIES

order which experience shows to be that of their general frequency in use.

A. The method devised by Strohl since the beginning of the war depends upon the proposition that in an isosceles triangle a vertical line from the apex bisects the base. Given such a triangle with the base equal to one-half its vertical altitude, then no matter how much the sides may be shortened or elongated, the base will maintain the same proportion, that is, will be equal to one-half of the altitude.

The apparatus is any table with an x-ray transparent top, with a tube in a box underneath so arranged that it may be made to travel in one line. Near the diaphragm of the tube box, and parallel to the table, is placed a card (z, Fig. 40) or other x-ray transparent medium. The distance from this card to the focus-spot of the tube is *carefully* measured, and the emergence of the vertical ray *carefully* marked on the card with a point (C), and through this point is drawn a line parallel to the excursion of the tube box. At right angles to this line are fixed (permanently) two wires so placed that each is at a distance from the central point C equal to one-fourth of the distance from C to the focus F. In other words, the two wires a and b are separated from each other by a distance equal to one-half the distance FC.

128 TREATMENT OF WAR WOUNDS

There is therefore a fixed isosceles triangle **F***ab* with a base *ab* and an altitude in the vertical line **FC**.

Use: Place on the table the part containing the projectile P and, with contracted diaphragm, cast

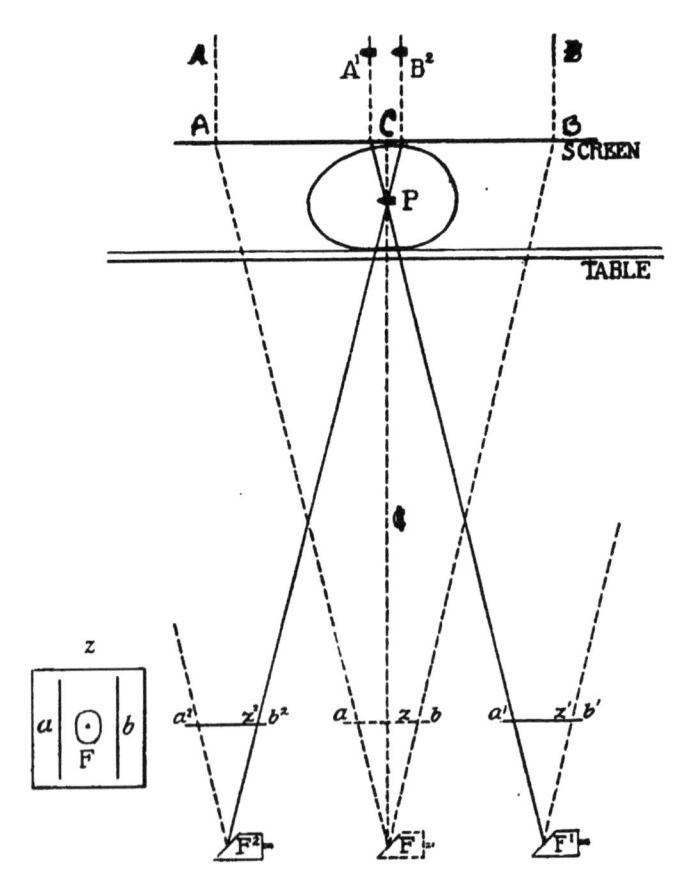

Fig. 40.—Diagram to illustrate method A.

the shadow of the projectile on the screen. A small hole in the screen is made to coincide with the shadow of the projectile. The skin is then marked through this hole. While this central tube position is maintained it may be found that the shadows of a and b are too widely separated to fall upon the screen. If, however, the tube is made to travel slowly to the right (F^1), the shadow A (of the wire a) will be seen to travel toward the shadow P (the shadow P meantime traveling almost imperceptibly toward A), and to finally coincide with it at a chosen point, say its middle A^1. This point is marked on the screen. The tube is then made to travel to the left (position F^2) until shadows B and P similarly coincide at B^2. The distance between A^1 and B^2 can now be measured on the screen and will be one-half the distance from the screen to the projectile. The army equipment contains a sliding scale for recording this distance without calculations. To find the distance from the skin to the projectile the distance between the skin and the screen (if they are not in contact) must be deducted. The depth reading should, in all cases, be supplemented by expert information, which can only be given by a properly trained observer, as to the anatomic position. Also, it would be desirable to have some indication or statement whereby the position of the part may be reproduced at the time of operation and the surgeon might find it desirable to attend a sufficient number of localizations by this and other methods to enable him clearly to understand what was actually done. This may well be supplemented, whenever opportunity permits, by inviting the roentgenologist to attend operations, to the end that he and the surgeon may become mutually helpful.

B. The second method utilizes the optical principle of parallax; that, given a plane surface, an object, and a movable light, the movement of the shadow will be proportionate to the distance of the object from the shadow surface (or toward the light). With two such moving shadows the shadow of the one nearest to the surface will move more slowly than that of the other farther away.

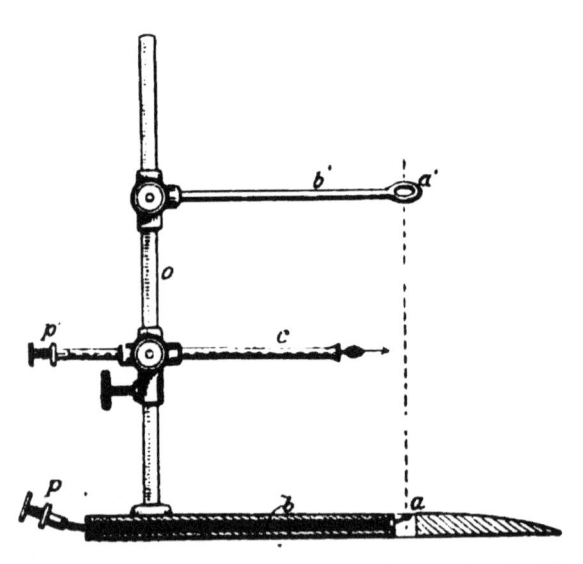

Fig. 41.—Diagram of army localizer. Applicable to method B and others.

In the army apparatus (Fig. 41) b is an aluminum base specially designed for being placed beneath the patient. a is an opening in that base. b' is a rod adjustable up and down an upright o and having an opening a' directly over a. The instrument is now shifted so that the foreign body shadow falls in the line a–a'. The opening in the pierced screen is also shifted to this line, and the skin is marked through the ring a'. With the aid of an inked plunger, p, the skin is also marked at a.

We have so far proceeded as in method a or b. Recourse is now had to c, a rod adjustable up and down and in and out on the upright o, also carrying an inked plunger, p'. A parallel ruling is laid upon the screen and the tube is shifted backward and forward (any convenient distance) and the rod c raised or lowered until its shadow and that of the foreign body have the same excursion. c is therefore at the same level as the foreign body and the skin is marked at this point. The instrument is now removed, and the distance of the foreign body from a or a' to c is readily determined by the provided adjustable scale.

C. In the third method the emergence of the central ray passing through the projectile is marked on the skin through the pierced screen, as in method A. A scale with parallel ruling of measured spaces is placed over the screen and the tube is moved until the shadow of the foreign body is intersected by one of these rulings. The shadow excursion is thus measured. This may be represented by diagram Fig. 42, in which s is the screen, t the table, f the focus, p the projectile, *1* and *2* the tube excursion, and *1'* and *2'* the shadow excursion.

In the army apparatus the distance ft is fixed, ts is measurable by a sliding scale, *1* to *2* by another

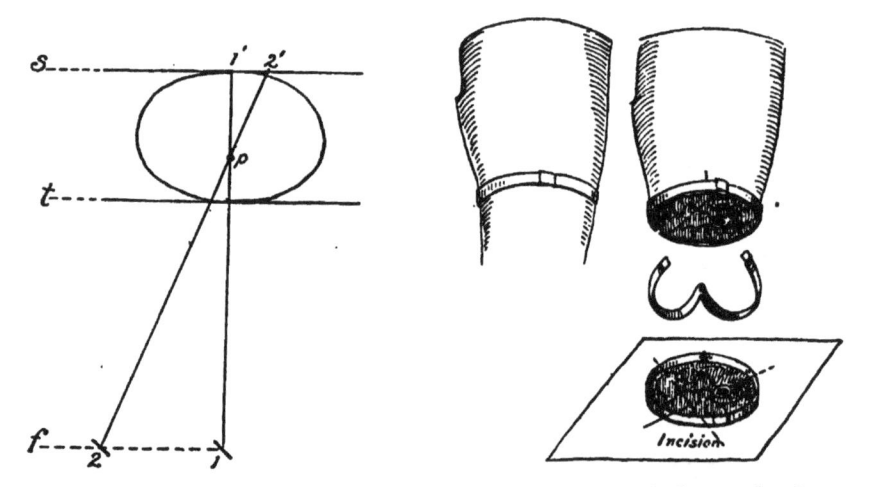

Fig. 42.—Diagram of method C.   Fig. 43.—The use of the profondometer
p, Projectile.   (Flint).

slider on the same scale, and *1'* to *2'* by the above described ruling (method B). It now only remains to transfer this to a standard diagram in which the line *1–1'* and the line s may be permanently laid out on the side wall and the points *2–2'* transferred from the sliding scale and connected by a thread. The distance *p–1'* is thus determined.

LOCALIZATION OF FOREIGN BODIES 133

These three methods, A, B, and C, are all fluoroscopic, require no arithmetic, as worked out for the army, and may be used according to the individual preference of the operator.

D. In this method, usually known as the "profondometer" (Fig. 43), use is made of flexible metal bands or of strips at right angles to each other which may be made to conform reasonably well to the body in the plane containing the foreign body. It involves the determination of at least two, and preferably three, lines of sight passing through the projectile and indicated by skin-marks. After the patient is removed from the fluoroscopic room, the assistant adjusts the flexible metal, which is made in two strips hinged together, so as to conform to the body in the plane of the skin-marks, transfers these marks to the metal so formed, carefully removes the metal without distortion, traces the body shape on a sheet of paper, and registers the skin-marks. These marks are suitably connected by straight lines. The intersection of these lines marks the position of the projectile with reference to the anatomic cross-section. If this is now compared with an anatomic cross-section of that particular region, the anatomic localization is quite definitely shown (Fig. 44). It is also possible, in some cases, to use a small in-

134 TREATMENT OF WAR WOUNDS

dicating rod and a flexible holder form to fit the body as a surgical indicator at the time of operation. This general method has been described in detail by Major Joseph Flint, M.R.C., and used quite satisfactorily by several surgeons.*

E. Of all the numerous indicating devices, compasses, etc., the one most generally accepted as useful

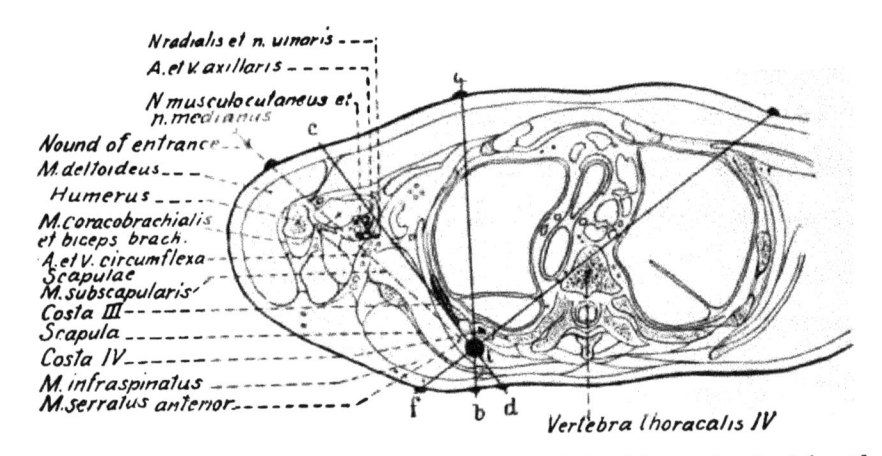

Fig. 44.—Profondometer outline of thorax and shoulder at level of fourth thoracic vertebra with structures sketched in and showing projectile anterior to internal border of scapula. *a, b, c, d, f,* etc., skin marks transferred to the chart by the profondometer, these marks being previously determined by methods A, B, or C. Elaborate detail in charts is not necessary in practice.

to the surgeon is the compass of Hirtz, or method "E" in the official list (Fig. 45). The roentgenologist must first determine by another method the depth of the foreign body from some convenient skin-point; second, he must then mark the skin at this

*Ann. Surg., Aug., 1916; Military Surgeon, March, 1917.

LOCALIZATION OF FOREIGN BODIES 135

point. Then, at each of three other suitably selected points on the skin, are to be attached small metallic markers, opaque to the rays. He must then determine the projection by vertical lines of these three markers and of the foreign body upon a plane surface, either on the fluoroscopic screen or the photo-

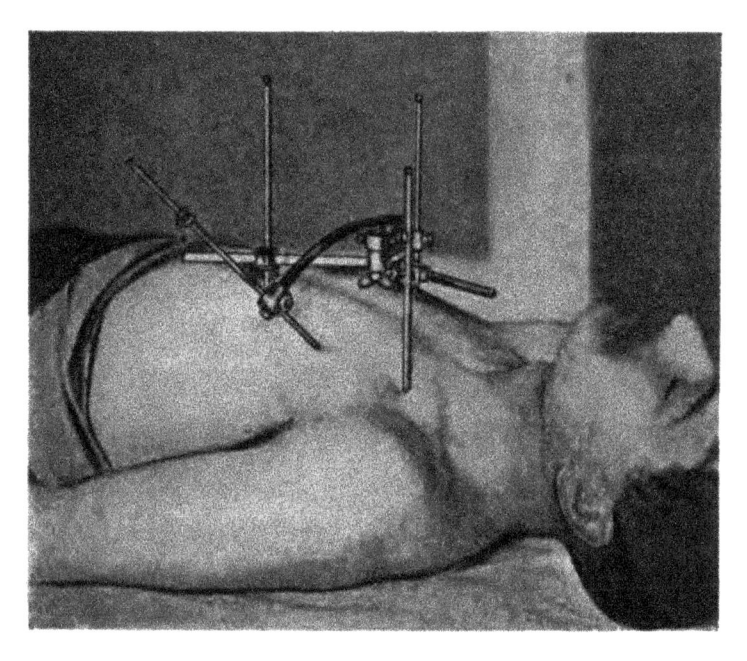

Fig. 45.—The Hirtz compass as applied to the patient at operation.

graphic plate. The next step is to determine the distance from that plane to the three markers, as well as to the foreign body. From these data a properly instructed assistant can so adjust the legs of the compass that, when placed upon the three selected skin-points, the indicating rod of the compass will point to the foreign body for any position of the arc or of the slider attached thereto, and will also register the depth along its own direction when the pointer touches the skin. Clearly, then, the advantage of this instrument to the surgeon is, first, that it furnishes a great number of definite sight lines from the exterior of the body to the projectile, and for each of these sight lines the proper depth. Second, the surgeon may select his point of incision and check his work at any time during the operation, provided the skin-marks are not displaced by the incision.

It cannot be said that, from a geometric standpoint, the Hirtz compass gives a more accurate localization than can be secured by other methods; in fact, it does not determine the initial localization, but it utilizes a simple depth in one direction to indicate a great number of depths each in a definite direction, and shows them in the simplest and most intelligible form for the use of the surgeon in the operating room.

While the detailed instruction is too elaborate for the scope of this article, the actual use of the method is very practical.

F. The last of the methods approved for use, but in which a very considerable degree of caution is advised, is the method of cannula and trocar, in which, under fluoroscopic control, a small trocar and cannula are pushed into the tissue until the instrument comes in contact with the projectile; the trocar (or obturator) is removed, and there is inserted a small wire with a barb at its distal end which attaches itself to tissue in the immediate vicinity of the foreign body and remains in place when the instrument is withdrawn, thus affording a direct guide to the projectile for the use of the surgeon. There are doubtless some advantages in this method, but it is advised that it be utilized only by experienced operators, and even then that care be taken to use it only where the danger of damage to important anatomic structures is a minimum.

Fluoroscopic Assistance During Operation.—Several methods have been proposed to utilize the fluoroscope at the time of operation, especially where the mobility of the projectile in the tissue or uncertainty of its position is such as to delay unduly the work of the surgeon.

The following extract from the report of the chief of the x-Ray Division of the American Expeditionary Force in France indicates the preparation which will be made for this class of work:

"The ordinary base hospital or portable table regularly furnished by the x-Ray Division of the

138   TREATMENT OF WAR WOUNDS

Surgeon General's Department of the army will serve admirably for this type of surgery, either operating with the bonnet fluoroscope in the usual bright light of the operating room, or by artificial

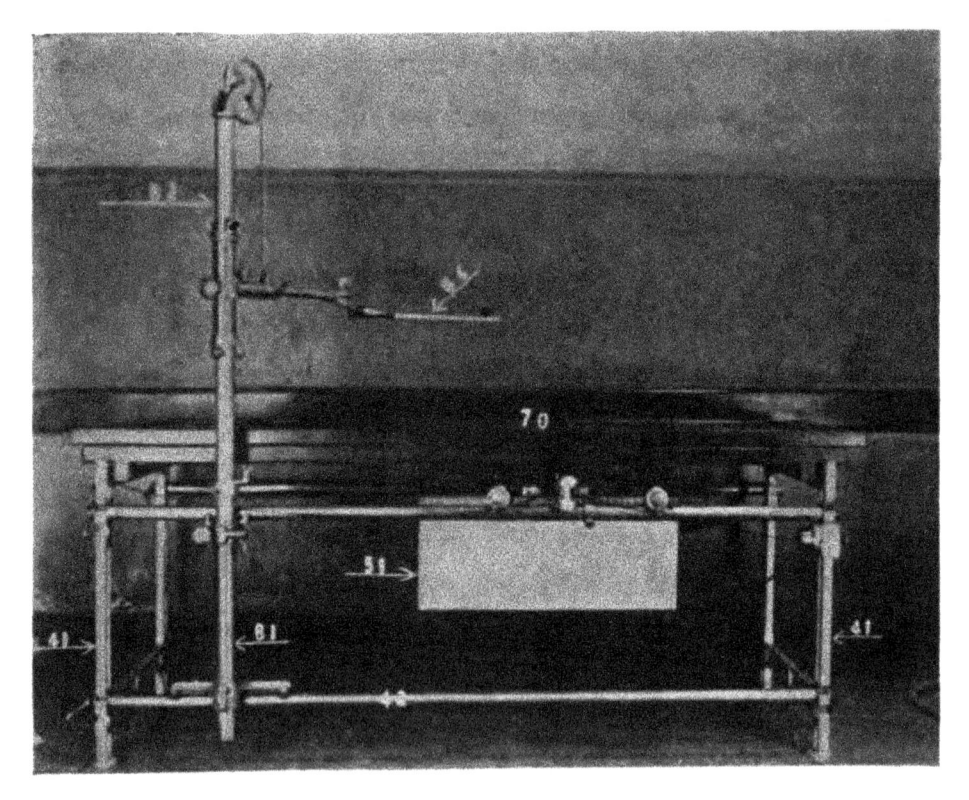

Fig. 46.—United States Army localizing table (numbers correspond to Localization Manual). 51, Movable protected tube box. 70, Transparent (to x-ray) table top. 84, Fluorescent screen (pierced).

light of suitable color in the fluoroscopic room of the x-Ray Department, with suitable arrangements for conveniently extinguishing the artificial light and turning on the current going to the x-ray tube. An order has been placed for extra base hospital tables without the screen supporting upright arm, to be issued to operating-rooms for this very purpose, our anticipation being that the bonnet method will be far more popular than the open screen method. We have acquired in France a small supply of collapsible operating tables with aluminum tops, also designed for this special type of radio-surgical work. Lacking any of these tables, the roentgenologist will be able to improvise a suitable equipment by combining the bedside outfit with an ordinary stretcher resting on the regular stretcher supports which will be available in the field.

"It is anticipated that the usual arrangement will be a base hospital table (without screen support) with overhead wire connections from the neighboring x-ray room, or there may be provided a special bedside unit, without a tube stand, to be used with a tube under the table.

"For operations in the usual light of the operating room there will be needed a bonnet fluoroscope so arranged that when the roentgenologist is not actually working with the x-ray, his accommodation will be preserved by means of dark glasses which are automatically dropped before his eyes when the hood of the bonnet fluoroscope is turned up; a special *metal pointer* (indicateur) for the roentgenologist, one for the surgeon, and a special forceps for projectile extracting, of special design, to protect the hands of the surgeon from the *x*-rays. A *foot switch* will be a help, but in the absence of one, an assistant can turn the current on or off at will. Both the hands of the roentgenologist will be in use, so that he may be free to work."

Stereofluoroscopy.—One of the principal difficulties in the localization of a foreign body arises from the fact that what is seen in the fluoroscopic and radiographic plate is simply a shadow projection which gives a fairly accurate idea of two dimensions in planes parallel to the plate or screen, but no visual evidence of relative position along the line of sight; that is, perpendicular to the plane of the receiving screen.

It has, of course, been possible for many years to do stereoscopic roentgenography. Two plates are taken in the same relative position in respect to the patient, but with a shift of the tube corresponding to the interpupillary distance, and these, with proper viewing devices, give a stereoscopic effect similar to that of the ordinary hand stereoscope.

Davidson worked out a method of utilizing two tubes, or of two targets in the same tube, by means of which stereoscopic fluoroscopy could be made possible.

Probably the most successful attempt to perfect this apparatus has recently been made by Major E. W. Caldwell, M.R.C., U.S.A., of New York, and while at the time of writing this apparatus has had only a laboratory test, it offers promise of becoming a very valuable addition to the apparatus now in use, especially where it is desirable to carry on an operation under fluoroscopic control.

The following description is taken from the article by Major Caldwell in the first edition of this work:

"With the ordinary fluoroscopic method, which gives no perception of depth, it is rather difficult to tell when the needle is approaching the foreign body. The stereofluoroscope, however, shows the relation of the exploring needle to the foreign body as accurately as it could be seen if exposed in the open air.

"The process of obtaining a stereo-fluoroscopic image is much more complicated than that of a simple fluoroscopy, but recent improvements in the x-ray tubes have removed many of the difficulties which existed in the first experiments some fifteen or eighteen years ago.

"In order to obtain the stereo-fluoroscopic image it is necessary to use two sources of x-ray, separated by a distance of a few inches, and to present to each eye the simple flat projection produced on the screen by one of these sources of x-ray. This is accomplished by exciting alternately the two sources (ordinarily two small tubes placed side by side) and moving in front of the eyes a shutter which is synchronous with the alternations in the source, so that when the right eye sees the projection from the left x-ray tube, the shutter cuts off the vision of the left eye. Conversely, when the left eye sees the projection from the right-hand x-ray tube, the shutter cuts off the view from the right eye. Each eye, therefore, sees a slightly different projection, and the effect is that of two-eye vision, which gives a conception of depth that is not obtained from the simple fluoroscopic shadow.

"In practice the flashes of the x-ray from each tube must follow each other so rapidly that the resulting x-ray shadow appears to be continuous. This requires a frequency of at least 15 or 16 impulses per second, and it is often convenient to use as many as 60 per second, which is the frequency of the usual commercial alternating current lighting circuit.

"My own first contribution to the art consisted in the use of a single tube with separated foci, and in the use of an electrically operated shutter, which was, therefore, freely movable and could be attached to the eye-piece of the ordinary fluoroscope. The alternating excitations of the tube were obtained by making use of an alternating current. The wave in one direction excited one source of x-ray, and the wave in the other direction excited the other source of x-ray. The moving shutter formed the rotor of a small synchronous electric motor operated from the same alternating current circuit which supplied current for the x-ray tube. At the present time this is the most convenient shutter available.

"In the last few years the development of the Coolidge tube, which can be operated perfectly from a high-tension alternating current, has made this problem very much simpler.

"Improved methods of supporting the tubes, the fluorescent screen, and the shutter have been developed within the last few months, and it is hoped that in spite of its complexity the apparatus may materially assist in the surgical removal of foreign bodies."

In Makins' paper[*] he and Major Curtis consider quite fully the use of radioscopy and stereo-fluoroscopy. They include also a consideration of the method of localization of foreign bodies by combining radiography and sectional anatomy, as described by Captain Crymble.[†] See also another important paper by Eastman and Bettman.[‡]

Hickey[§] urges the employment of the x-ray stereoscopic views, taken *transversely* across the body.

[*] Brit. Med. Jour., June 16, 1917.
[†] Brit. Jour. Surg., October, 1915.
[‡] Annals of Surgery, July, 1917.
[§] Amer. Jour. Roentgenol., March, 1917.

REMOVAL OF FOREIGN BODIES

If the foreign body is removed, it is desirable, as Webb and Mulligan point out, *to show it to the patient*, as it has an excellent moral effect upon him.

The ordinary surgical instruments for extracting such foreign bodies are always available.

Rayner and Barclay (Brit. Med. Jour., February 23, 1918) describe a very ingenious extractor by which they succeeded in extracting a small foreign body from the brain by alternately using daylight and a fluorescent screen with the x-rays.

In a number of cases very powerful magnets have been used in the removal of metallic foreign bodies made of iron or steel. Those made of lead, copper, etc., are not amenable to this treatment (*vide* Cushing's experience, p. 198).

A vibrator actuated by coarse alternations of the electric current may loosen such a foreign body.

TETANUS

The infection of the soil and of the skin and clothes, the sealing of the wounds from drying of the blood when speedy access to the first-aid station is impossible, so creating an anaërobic condition in the wound, the rapid growth of the bacteria in twenty-four hours or more in such favorable conditions, all combined to cause many cases of tetanus in the early months of the war. In our Civil War the mortality was 89.3 per cent.; in the Franco-Prussian War, 90 per cent. Ashhurst and John,* in a paper covering 435 cases from 1897–1911, reported by 13 authors, still showed a mortality of 60 per cent. In the early stages of the present war there were necessarily many cases, because of lack of the tetanus antitoxin in sufficient quantities for such huge masses of wounded. By November, 1914, the supply became sufficient and the mortality immediately dropped. At the beginning of the war, too, the imperative need of an early protective inoculation had not been driven deep into the minds of surgeons, as has been the case later.

* Amer. Jour. Med. Sci., June, 1913.

Now every wounded man receives a protective inoculation at the very first possible moment. As Gibson insists, to wait for the symptoms of trismus is to court disaster. "Expect tetanus in all wounds and prevent its onset" is the rule, and the result has been that lockjaw has almost disappeared in the armies on both sides. This conquest of tetanus is one of the notable victories of the war.

Sir David Bruce has made a careful study of 1000 cases of tetanus in the base hospitals in England.* Including the cases in France not transferred to England, he estimates the percentage of cases at 0.2 per cent. Of the 1000 cases, 896 were of the usual general type, 99 were localized, and 5 were doubtful. In "localized tetanus" only the muscles in the neighborhood of the wound are involved. All these local cases recovered. (*Vide* pp. 153 and 160.)

The shorter the period of incubation, the greater was the mortality. Happily the number of the acute cases with short incubation periods has steadily diminished as the war progressed. In one case this incubation period was as long as one hundred and ninety days.

Of the 1000 cases, 594 recovered and 406 died, a mortality rate of 40.6 per cent. If we include the

* Brit. Med. Jour., February 23, 1918.

cases which remained in France, the mortality is probably 50 per cent. But in the pre-antitoxin days it was 85 to 90 per cent. The number of cases also was enormous. The gain, both in the smaller number of cases and of deaths, is exceedingly great. After Waterloo Sir Charles Bell wrote, "there are but two cases living of all that had this affection!" In Bruce's five successive partial reports of the English cases the mortality which began at 57.7 per cent. fell steadily, series by series, to 49.2 per cent., 36.5 per cent., 31 per cent., and in the last series in 1917 to 19 per cent. Among the 1000 cases 40 cases did *not* receive the antitoxin, and 32, *80 per cent.*, died. In the 960 cases which *had* received the antitoxin, the mortality was only *38.8 per cent.*

"*Antitoxin has no power of neutralizing toxin fixed in the nervous system. If a fatal amount has been absorbed, then no amount of antitoxin will save the man's life.*"

The inference is plain. The patient should receive the antitoxin at the *very earliest moment possible*, so as to *prevent this fatal absorption.*

One peculiar phase of infection has been noted by Moynihan and others, viz., "the inordinate length of time microörganisms may remain in the tissues long after healing is complete" and then cause acute infection. *Even after trivial operations* for the removal of foreign bodies, or even for passive movements, tetanus may set in unexpectedly. "Delayed tetanus" and "delayed gas infection" are not very uncommon.

Bowling* records three instructive cases under treatment at one time, delayed until the fortieth, fifty-first, and fifty-third days. In the forty-day case not only did tetanus set in after this period, but seventy-three days after the wound had been received, and forty-two days after it had healed, gas gangrene also supervened and caused his death. Meantime his tetanus had yielded after the administration of a total of 189,500 units. No operative interference had occurred to light up these two infections. The other two cases had received antitetanic injections—one at an uncertain interval, the other two days after being wounded. Probably none had been given to the first (the fatal) case. Both of the other cases followed slight operations— one sixteen days after the mere opening of an abscess, the other four days after the removal of some clothing and part of the casing of a bullet.

In animals anaphylaxis following a second injection of the same serum is well known. But in man this is much less to be feared. Still, provision should be

* Brit. Med. Jour., March 4, 1916, p. 337.

made to prevent its occurrence. It may follow a second dose of the antitetanic serum when this is given at an interval of ten to twelve days after the first dose. If, therefore, ten or twelve days after the prophylactic dose of the serum has been given, tetanus is threatened, the serum should be administered in fractional doses as follows: Instead of a full dose, an injection of only two or three drops of the serum in solution should be given; if no ill results follow within ten minutes more, the full dose may then be administered. Fractional doses should be the rule *when any operations*—even minor ones, such as described above—have to be done after an interval of ten to twelve days. If shock should occur, a few minims of a 1 : 1000 solution of adrenalin may be given hypodermically if the shock is not severe, but intravenously if it is at all alarming.

I append the Memorandum on Tetanus issued by the British War Office Committee on the Study of Tetanus: The necessity of several successive protective doses is properly emphasized.

Memorandum on Tetanus

Third Edition, June, 1917 *

"*The Prophylactic or Preventive Treatment of Tetanus.*—The prophylactic value of injections of antitetanic serum is beyond all question, but there is strong experimental evidence that in about ten days the immunity conferred by the primary injection is to a great extent lost.

"It is impossible, from the appearance of any wound, to determine whether it is infected with tetanus bacilli or not; and whereas many cases of tetanus have occurred not only in men with healed wounds, but also in those whose wounds were from the beginning practically clean, it has been decided that all wounded men shall receive at least *four* injections of antitetanic serum; that is to say, a primary injection given at the time of the wound and three others.

"It is, therefore, essential that a second, third, and fourth subcutaneous injection should be given to all wounded men, and in order to anticipate the total disappearance of antitoxin from the body, the second injection should follow the first at an interval of seven days, or as soon after this as possible. The third and fourth injections must also follow at the same interval of time.

* Received through the courtesy of Dr. Dawson Williams, Editor of the British Medical Journal.

"As many cases of tetanus have occurred in men suffering from trench feet, sometimes without obvious breach of surface, these cases must be treated as wounded men.

"It may be definitely stated here that the danger of anaphylactic shock is negligible when prophylactic doses of 500 U. S. A. units contained in 3 cm. of horse serum are given subcutaneously, whatever the interval after the preceding injection. . . .

"*Dosage in Prophylactic or Preventive Treatment of Tetanus.*—The primary injection should consist of 500 U. S. A. units, and the second, third, and fourth injections should be of the same amount.

"The primary injection is given, as a rule, at a dressing station or field ambulance as soon as the wounded soldier is removed from the firing line. The second and following injections will most frequently be given at home hospitals. . . . The ordinary phial usually contains 1500 units of tetanus antitoxin. One-third of a phial should, therefore, be injected into each wounded man. Phials containing 500 units are also now available. There is no necessity to sterilize the syringes after each injection—the serum is aseptic, and, moreover, contains an antiseptic; it will be sufficient if a freshly sterilized needle is used for each case. Care should be taken to insure that the skin and needle are both sterilized, as neglect of this precaution is apt to lead to abscess formation.

"*Precautions to be Taken Before Operating on Wounds.—When operations are performed at the site of wounds, even if they are healed, a prophylactic injection of serum should invariably be given if the operation be performed at a greater interval than seven days from the last injection. This precaution is very necessary as numerous cases have occurred in which the performance of a simple operation has been followed by an attack of tetanus, although in many cases the primary wound had been healed several weeks before the operation.*

"*This precautionary injection may consist of a single subcutaneous injection of the ordinary prophylactic dose of 500 units. Of course, a larger dose than 500 units may be injected if thought advisable.*

"It is better to give it two days before the operation, as it takes some forty-eight hours for the antitoxin to be fully absorbed after subcutaneous injection. Injected intramuscularly, the absorption is quicker,—probably in about twelve hours,—so that this method could be used if time is pressing.

"*Antiseptics Which May be of Use in the Preventive Treatment of Tetanus.*—The group of oxidizing antiseptics, such as hydrogen peroxid, potassium permanganate, chlorin water, Dakin's solution, and solution of iodin, are particularly unfavorable to the anaërobic growth of the tetanus bacillus. They have the power of rendering toxin non-toxic.

"*Diagnosis.*—The classic symptoms of tetanus as described in the majority of the text-books refer to a phase of the disease in which treatment will have lost much of its power and value. With many medical men tetanus is not tetanus until the symptoms of *risus* sardonicus and lockjaw are present.

"In those who have been partially protected by a prophylactic injection of antitoxin, trismus and general symptoms may not occur at all or not until late in the disease, possibly not until months have elapsed. This is known as '*delayed tetanus.*' In such cases the manifestations of tetanus may be confined to local spastic rigidity of the wounded limb, which may persist for weeks or months and then disappear, or may be developed into generalized tetanus. This so-called '*localized tetanus*' is a distinct and not infrequent type of the disease and should be carefully watched for.

"*The early diagnosis of tetanus is of the greatest importance. All clinical and experimental evidence tends to show that the chances of successful treatment diminish rapidly as the length of time increases after the first symptoms have been observed.*

"**Tetanus toxin reaches the motor nerve-cells of the central nervous system by traveling up the nerves. It is not directly conveyed to the nerve-cells by the blood.** In a large number of cases the toxin appears to reach the spinal cord primarily by the nerves which are in connection with the seat of the injury, and hence the motor nerve-cells governing the muscles around about the wound will be the earliest affected, such affection showing itself in the form of spasticity and increased reflex excitability of these muscles. The patient may complain of jerking or jumping, or stiffness in the affected limb, occurring especially at night. In some cases these symptoms may precede the other symptoms of tetanus by many hours or days. It is, therefore, desirable that the muscles in the vicinity of the wound should be examined whenever dressings are removed, and the occurrence of rigidity or twitchings, or local increased reflex response to gentle tapping or pressure should be immediately reported to the surgeon in charge.

"*All nursing sisters engaged in dressing wounds should be warned to give the alarm if the muscles around the wound should be harder or more rigid than the muscles of the uninjured limb or side.*

"In other cases tetanus toxin is absorbed from the wound into the blood-stream and reaches the central nervous system by way of nerves other than those in direct anatomic continuity with the wound, and, hence, early symptoms may sometimes be observed in muscles supplied by any motor segment of the cord or brain.

"The muscles supplied by the fifth nerve are those most commonly affected, as is shown by the occurrence of trismus as an early symptom. In a wounded man this symptom should be taken as a decisive indication of tetanus in the absence of any other obvious source of reflex spasm. Other cranial nerve symptoms may be facial spasm or paralysis, or paralysis or spasm of the eye muscles with consequent strabismus.

"Spasm of the pharyngeal muscles may also occur,

which is often complained of by the patient as sore throat, and occasionally causes reflex yawning. The tongue muscles may be affected, causing deviation of the tongue when protruded. Tetanic spasm of the neck muscles may be complained of as stiff neck. Spasm of the thoracic and abdominal muscles is an occasional early symptom, often giving rise to complaints of stitch in the side or to difficulty in micturition.

"Often before the onset of any definite symptom of tetanus there is a general increase of muscular tone, and the deep reflexes are exaggerated; knee and ankle clonus may be produced in the absence of any signs pointing to the involvement of the pyramidal tract, such as an extensor plantar response or loss of the abdominal reflexes.

"The general increase of tone is manifested in the facial muscles by the drawn expression of the patient, and the increased reflex excitability often leads to psychical irritability and insomnia.

"The occurrence of a generalised tetanic toxemia may be marked by profuse local or generalised sweating.

"Once the diagnosis of tetanus has been definitely established, the patient should be examined as little as possible.

"*Therapeutic or Curative Treatment of Tetanus.—It cannot be too strongly emphasized that time is the all-important element in the treatment of tetanus. As short a time as possible should be allowed to elapse be-*

tween the diagnosis and the commencement of active treatment. A delay of an hour may make all the difference between success and failure.

"It is on this account that the early symptoms are of the greatest importance. In almost every case of tetanus there are found local manifestations of the disease, very often hardness and rigidity of the muscles around the wound, and these signs can be seen or felt for days or even weeks before the occurrence of trismus. In a case on record these local symptoms had been present for three weeks before the trismus showed itself and before tetanus was suspected. One medical officer is reported to have said that symptoms of tetanus were present in a case but were not sufficiently severe to justify the use of antitoxin! According to present ideas, it should no longer be permissible to wait for the occurrence of lockjaw before deciding that the case is [one of] tetanus; 5000 units of antitoxic serum are of more avail at the very beginning, when the disease is still localized, than 50,000 when the symptoms have become general. The moment, then, that *any* local manifestation of tetanus is observed, it is recommended to proceed at once to vigorous specific treatment.

"The treatment of tetanus may be divided into specific and symptomatic:

"I. Specific.—Specific treatment consists in the giving of tetanus antitoxin, which has the power of neutralizing the tetanus toxin with which it comes in contact. The problem in treatment is to bring about this contact in the fullest and speediest manner. There are four methods which are commonly employed for the administration of antitoxin:

"(a) *Subcutaneous.*—In this method the serum is injected beneath the skin, from whence it is slowly absorbed into the circulation; it has been determined that some forty-eight hours elapse before the maximum concentration in the blood is reached. This slowness of absorption is an advantage when it is desired that the action of the serum should be prolonged, as in prophylactic administration. But it is a grave disadvantage when quickness of action is all-important, as in acute tetanus; in such a case little can be expected from this method at the beginning of treatment, although it is useful later in order to keep up the antitoxic action.

"(b) *Intramuscular.*—Here the serum is injected into the muscles, from which it is absorbed into the circulation more rapidly than from the subcutaneous tissues. It is, therefore, as regards speed, better than the subcutaneous method: nevertheless, it must be remembered that full absorption, even here, takes twelve or more hours.

"(c) *Intravenous.*—Here the serum is injected directly into the blood-stream and immediately diffused throughout the body in such a way as to neutralize all circulating toxin. This is the most rapid route by which the neutralization of circulating toxin can be accomplished. The objection to this method is that large doses of serum introduced into

the circulation, in persons who have previously had an injection, is apt to bring about anaphylactic shock, which may prove fatal. Intravenous injection is, therefore, not recommended except in cases where the intrathecal method is, for any reason, impossible.

"(d) *Intrathecal.*—Here the serum is introduced by lumbar puncture into the subarachnoid space of the spinal canal. It soon begins to escape into the bloodstream, so that the neutralization of circulating toxin is quickly effected.

"*The Committee is of opinion that in acute general tetanus the best method of treatment lies in the earliest possible administration of large doses of antitoxic serum by the intrathecal route, repeated on two, three, or four days in succession, and combined, if thought desirable, with intramuscular injections.*

"The introduction of the serum into the subarachnoid space always produces turbidity of the cerebrospinal fluid, due to polymorphonuclear leukocytosis; this reaction is sometimes associated with transient symptoms of meningeal irritation, which need cause no alarm. With ordinary precautions the risk of septic infection is negligible.

"In the *chronic forms of tetanus*, particularly the form of localized tetanus limited to one limb, without trismus or other sign of generalization, there appears to be no need to resort to intrathecal injection. A course of serum treatment by the intramuscular method will, in most cases, do all that is required.

"*Dosage in the Therapeutic or Curative Treatment of Tetanus.—Experience has shown that in the treatment of acute general tetanus the best results are obtained from very large doses of serum; the more acute the case the larger should be the doses of serum employed.* The object is to saturate the body with antitoxin as quickly as possible and to maintain the saturation. For this purpose from 50,000 to 100,000 units may be given during the first few days of treatment.

"Tetanus antitoxin is issued to military hospitals in two strengths. The weaker is put up in phials containing either 500 or 1500 units, the more concentrated in phials containing 8000 units. Every general hospital should have in stock a supply of the high potency serum in order that there may be no delay should a case of acute tetanus occur in the district. This high potency serum should always be employed for intrathecal injections, because this route differs from the others in the fact that the amount of fluid which can be introduced is limited. This high potency serum should be reserved for intrathecal injections alone.

"The amount of cerebrospinal fluid which can be withdrawn on lumbar puncture will not, as a rule, be more than 20 c.c. It is usually held to be undesirable to run in more serum than will replace the cerebrospinal fluid drawn off, and in cases when little or no fluid can be withdrawn it is not wise to inject more than 20 c.c. of serum, *and this very slowly.* The 16,000 units, contained in two phials of the high

the circulation, in persons who have previously had an injection, is apt to bring about anaphylactic shock, which may prove fatal. Intravenous injection is, therefore, not recommended except in cases where the intrathecal method is, for any reason, impossible.

"(d) *Intrathecal.*—Here the serum is introduced by lumbar puncture into the subarachnoid space of the spinal canal. It soon begins to escape into the bloodstream, so that the neutralization of circulating toxin is quickly effected.

"*The Committee is of opinion that in acute general tetanus the best method of treatment lies in the earliest possible administration of large doses of antitoxic serum by the intrathecal route, repeated on two, three, or four days in succession, and combined, if thought desirable, with intramuscular injections.*

"The introduction of the serum into the subarachnoid space always produces turbidity of the cerebrospinal fluid, due to polymorphonuclear leukocytosis; this reaction is sometimes associated with transient symptoms of meningeal irritation, which need cause no alarm. With ordinary precautions the risk of septic infection is negligible.

"In the *chronic forms of tetanus*, particularly the form of localized tetanus limited to one limb, without trismus or other sign of generalization, there appears to be no need to resort to intrathecal injection. A course of serum treatment by the intramuscular method will, in most cases, do all that is required.

"*Dosage in the Therapeutic or Curative Treatment of Tetanus.*—Experience has shown that in the treatment of acute general tetanus the best results are obtained from very large doses of serum; the more acute the case the larger should be the doses of serum employed. The object is to saturate the body with antitoxin as quickly as possible and to maintain the saturation. For this purpose from 50,000 to 100,000 units may be given during the first few days of treatment.

"Tetanus antitoxin is issued to military hospitals in two strengths. The weaker is put up in phials containing either 500 or 1500 units, the more concentrated in phials containing 8000 units. Every general hospital should have in stock a supply of the high potency serum in order that there may be no delay should a case of acute tetanus occur in the district. This high potency serum should always be employed for intrathecal injections, because this route differs from the others in the fact that the amount of fluid which can be introduced is limited. This high potency serum should be reserved for intrathecal injections alone.

"The amount of cerebrospinal fluid which can be withdrawn on lumbar puncture will not, as a rule, be more than 20 c.c. It is usually held to be undesirable to run in more serum than will replace the cerebrospinal fluid drawn off, and in cases when little or no fluid can be withdrawn it is not wise to inject more than 20 c.c. of serum, *and this very slowly.* The 16,000 units, contained in two phials of the high

the circulation, in persons who have previously had an injection, is apt to bring about anaphylactic shock, which may prove fatal. Intravenous injection is, therefore, not recommended except in cases where the intrathecal method is, for any reason, impossible.

"(d) *Intrathecal.*—Here the serum is introduced by lumbar puncture into the subarachnoid space of the spinal canal. It soon begins to escape into the bloodstream, so that the neutralization of circulating toxin is quickly effected.

"*The Committee is of opinion that in acute general tetanus the best method of treatment lies in the earliest possible administration of large doses of antitoxic serum by the intrathecal route, repeated on two, three, or four days in succession, and combined, if thought desirable, with intramuscular injections.*

"The introduction of the serum into the subarachnoid space always produces turbidity of the cerebrospinal fluid, due to polymorphonuclear leukocytosis; this reaction is sometimes associated with transient symptoms of meningeal irritation, which need cause no alarm. With ordinary precautions the risk of septic infection is negligible.

"In the *chronic forms of tetanus*, particularly the form of localized tetanus limited to one limb, without trismus or other sign of generalization, there appears to be no need to resort to intrathecal injection. A course of serum treatment by the intramuscular method will, in most cases, do all that is required.

"*Dosage in the Therapeutic or Curative Treatment of Tetanus.—Experience has shown that in the treatment of acute general tetanus the best results are obtained from very large doses of serum; the more acute the case the larger should be the doses of serum employed. The object is to saturate the body with antitoxin as quickly as possible and to maintain the saturation. For this purpose from 50,000 to 100,000 units may be given during the first few days of treatment.*

"Tetanus antitoxin is issued to military hospitals in two strengths. The weaker is put up in phials containing either 500 or 1500 units, the more concentrated in phials containing 8000 units. Every general hospital should have in stock a supply of the high potency serum in order that there may be no delay should a case of acute tetanus occur in the district. This high potency serum should always be employed for intrathecal injections, because this route differs from the others in the fact that the amount of fluid which can be introduced is limited. This high potency serum should be reserved for intrathecal injections alone.

"The amount of cerebrospinal fluid which can be withdrawn on lumbar puncture will not, as a rule, be more than 20 c.c. It is usually held to be undesirable to run in more serum than will replace the cerebrospinal fluid drawn off, and in cases when little or no fluid can be withdrawn it is not wise to inject more than 20 c.c. of serum, *and this very slowly*. The 16,000 units, contained in two phials of the high be communicated to the officers and medical practitioners in charge of subsidiary hospitals. . . .

"On the occurrence of a case of tetanus the appointed officer will be immediately informed, and he will at once proceed to visit the case and offer assistance in the carrying out of such treatment as has been suggested in the present memorandum. He will, if necessary, assist in the operation of lumbar puncture and intrathecal injection. This will seldom be necessary, as from what has already been said as to the danger of even an hour's delay this intrathecal injection will usually have been given before his arrival. He will make careful inquiry into the case in order to ascertain if any early symptoms had been present and had escaped notice. He will note what prophylactic injections had been made, and if omitted, why they were omitted. When visiting the hospital where the case has occurred, he will ascertain if the other wounded men are receiving prophylactic injections. He should see that sufficient notes of the case are being kept in order that the tetanus form can be filled up as fully as possible. For example, it is very seldom that the distinguishing marks on the bottles of serum are reported. If serum trouble arises, it is evident that this information would be useful. He will forward an inspector's report to [the proper officer] with as little delay as possible. The ordinary tetanus report will be filled in by the medical officer in charge of the case. [In the United States Army this report would go to the surgeon's immediately superior officer unless other special orders had been issued.] Too great care cannot be taken in this matter of the reports, as the value of any analysis made from them depends on their accuracy and completeness.

"*Officers in charge of hospitals will be responsible for the administration of the second, third, and fourth prophylactic doses of antitoxin to all wounded under their care unless grave reasons exist for withholding them.*

"*When patients are transferred from one hospital to another the number of injections given, with the dates, must be entered on the* [history which will accompany the patient].

"On the death or recovery of the patient, they will forward the usual tetanus report in accordance with [the Surgeon General's] instructions.

"Any abnormalities of behavior of antitetanic serum should be carefully noted and reported.

"As the Tetanus Committee was appointed for the purpose of studying tetanus, it is greatly to be desired that every medical officer will coöperate in a collective investigation, and submit any evidence in his possession which may add to our knowledge of the disease and its treatment.

"*Instruction to Medical Officers in Charge of the Wounded.*—[Every medical officer in the field should be familiar with the foregoing instructions and be held responsible for carrying them out, especially by the first prophylactic injection. He 'should bear in mind that *cases of trench feet* are especially dangerous.' As soon as tetanus is suspected the patient should be removed to a special ward where light and sound can be excluded and placed under the care of a thoroughly trustworthy and sympathetic nurse."]

APPENDIX

The Method of Performing an Intrathecal Injection

"The patient should preferably be under general anesthesia. The skin over the area of the fourth and fifth lumbar spines should be painted with iodin or cleansed with soap and water, followed by an antiseptic. A spinal needle and 20 c.c. syringe should be boiled in normal saline, *and the surgeon must observe throughout the most rigorous aseptic precautions.*

"The patient is bent head to knees, so as to present as fully a curved back to the operator as possible, and the position of the fourth lumbar spine ascertained by drawing an imaginary line between the highest points of the crests of the ilia.

"The tip of the finger is placed on the supraspinous ligament connecting the summits of the spinous processes of the fourth and fifth lumbar vertebræ. The needle is inserted about three-eighths of an inch to one side of the middle line, and directed forward and slightly upward and inward. If the needle strikes the bone, it should be withdrawn and a fresh attempt made. The canal is reached at a depth, on an average, of about $2\frac{1}{2}$ inches (5 cm.). The trocar is withdrawn, and about 20 c.c. of cerebrospinal fluid allowed to flow out into a measured vessel. The syringe is then fitted to the needle and the serum injected.

"It is important that the serum be heated to the temperature of the body and the injection made very slowly.

"The canal can also be reached by pushing the needle through the supraspinous ligament in the middle line, half-way between the two spinous processes.

"If several injections have to be made, it is well to choose fresh sites.

"Blocking of the flow of the cerebrospinal fluid by a blood-clot may be overcome by reinserting and withdrawing the trocar.

"The bed should be tilted at the foot and the pillow removed for an hour or two after the injections."

GAS INFECTION AND GAS GANGRENE

e difference between these two conditions should
ticed.

s infection is very common in the wounded in
resent war. As Bowlby notes, it is practically
own in Great Britain. The same is true in the
ed States. Personally I never saw a single case
e Civil War, and but one case in civil life since
In the present war Taylor notes the presence
le gas bacillus of Welch in 70 per cent. of the
. Fleming* found it in 103 wounds out of 127,
n the clothing in 10 out of 12 cases. Fortunately
nfection can be controlled with much success if
seen and treated early.

s gangrene, on the contrary, is a result of pro-
ively developed infection and is a most dangerous
lition.

ne cause is most commonly the bacillus of Welch
aërogenes capsulatus, often called B. perfringens
:he French. Other gas-producing bacteria are
found.

* Lancet, September 18, 1915, p. 638.

The rapidity of the growth of the bacillus of Welch, and therefore the urgent need of instant and radical action, is best appreciated by Kenneth Taylor's method of obtaining a pure culture:* A series of six or more culture-tubes are inoculated, each tube from its predecessor, at intervals of only half an hour. Even in this short interval bubbles of gas become evident in the successive tubes. By the sixth or seventh tube one may obtain a pure culture, so far has the gas bacillus outgrown all other germs.

The bacteriologist and the surgeon should constantly coöperate, as so convincingly urged by Carrel.

Tissier's observations† are illuminating. Working on wounds in the present war, and by animal experimentation, he has shown the following noteworthy facts: Filtered cultures of the Welch bacillus and of that of malignant edema when injected into animals were inert. Unfiltered cultures were followed by only a hard edema, which gradually disappeared. If, however, there were added to the Welch bacillus various aërobic cultures, the death of the animal soon followed. If the added culture consisted of the enterococcus, then a guinea-pig would be killed in

* "Pathol. and Bact. of Gas Gangrene," Jour. Path. and Bact., 1916, xx, 384.

† Ann. Institut. Pasteur, December, 1916.

three days; if it were the staphylococcus albus, death followed in twenty-four hours; if the streptococcus was added, death followed in fifteen hours. This symbiosis of aërobic and anaërobic bacteria is of great biologic interest and of great practical importance. Bashford notes that this combination is "exceedingly virulent."

The marked difference between the action of a pure culture and a mixed culture Tissier attributes to the restraint on the anaërobes by the oxygen in the circulating blood. The observation of Bowlby that he has never seen gas gangrene in the head, and almost never in the neck, affords strong support to this view, as their blood-supply is far more abundant than that of any other part of the body. The addition of the aërobes removes this restraint. The latter, so to speak, prepare the soil and allow the anaërobes then to play their destructive rôle. For the first six to eight hours the wounds contain few bacteria; by the tenth hour the anaërobes begin to multiply rapidly; by twelve hours they are the dominant growth.

Clinically also the same astonishingly rapid development is seen. Bowlby* has observed well-marked infection with formation of gas within five hours,

* Brit. Jour. Surg., 1915–16, 151.

and death from gas gangrene of an entire limb in sixteen hours. In the long muscles the transition from mere tissue injury to wide-spread bacillary infection is marked. The part distal to the wound has its blood-supply cut off, especially by thrombosis. Histologic studies show that the products of the bacilli damage both the muscle-fibers and the blood-vessels ahead of the mass invasion. The bacilli may spread across the muscle in the track of the blood-vessels. "The bacteria get away easily into the muscular tissues from the cesspool of the wound and multiply enormously" (Bashford). In the part proximal to the wound the blood-supply is preserved, and this part suffers far less. The short segmented muscles, *e. g.*, the rectus abdominis, suffer much less than the long muscles.

All foreign bodies in the wound (especially clothing), as they will keep up the anaërobic infection, must be removed; *all* dead tissue must be removed. This complete removal of all dead muscular tissue is fundamental. The dirty brick-red color is one guide. Another is the contractility of the muscle. Parts which do not contract when severed by the knife are dead and must be sacrificed. Parts which do contract—and also *bleed*—are living and may be left. Not seldom an entire long muscle must be removed; sometimes an entire group. The wound must be kept open, and frequent antiseptic dressings used. My own impression is that Dakin's fluid, possibly Taylor's quinin chlorhydrate, and other antiseptics, when properly used in connection with the above absolutely necessary means, will enable the surgeon to conquer the infection at the start, *if he sees the patient early enough*—certainly within the first twenty-four hours. If the infection has gained headway and gas production has already set in, then the treatment by incisions and all means to facilitate the escape of the gas, and nothing which will hinder it, with further removal of dead tissue and the continued use of the chosen antiseptic, especially by Carrel's method, in many cases will result in cure. If gas gangrene has actually occurred, certainly if it is extensive, then immediate amputation will be needful in many, if not in most, cases.

The gas is produced by the destruction especially of the muscular tissue, and accumulates at first in and between the muscular bundles. A detached arm or leg will sometimes float in water because of the great quantity of gas in it. If a small puncture is made and a lighted match be applied, the gas will take fire and burn with a blue flame (Bashford). In the intramuscular spaces it quickly compresses the muscular tissues mechanically until it bursts the sheath. Meantime necrosis of the tissue occurs, and a severe toxemia may easily follow.

Treatment.—The paramount importance of the earliest possible treatment during the first stage of rapidly spreading infection, before the production of gas in any serious quantity has occurred, is self-evident. Every hour counts against the patient.

Taylor* points out clearly what is to be done:

1. Destruction of the bacillus.

2. Removal of the tissue especially favoring its growth, *i. e.*, the necrotic muscles.

3. Measures to prevent the destruction of the muscles as a result of mechanical pressure.

Thorough extirpation alone, especially, of course, if done early and in a segmented muscle, may be curative. Bashford† mentions a case of beginning gas gangrene of the rectus abdominis caused by a retained piece of shrapnel and a piece of an overcoat seven to nine square inches in size. The foreign bodies were removed, all the tissues surrounding them and the wound were excised, the wound was

* "La Gangrène Gazeuse," Arch. de méd. et de pharmacie militaire, 1916; Lancet, September 4, 1915, 538, and January 15, 1916, 123; Brit. Med. Jour., December 25, 1915, 923.

† Brit. Jour. Surg., 1916–17, iv, 568.

cleansed with simple sterile water and healed *per primam*. Yet the metal and the clothing were rich in bacteria, including the Welch bacillus. This excellent paper well repays careful perusal.

Should the antitoxin of Bull and Pritchett prove as valuable as is hoped for, the very first step should be the intravenous injection of the antitoxin; all the other measures may be used as adjuvants, but this is the sheet anchor.

For the destruction of the bacilli Taylor recommends a 1 per cent. solution of chlorhydrate of quinin. Others have found Dakin's fluid effective.

As the bacillus of Welch is an anaërobe, oxygen is inimical to its growth. Depage has used injections of oxygen into the tissues infected with the Welch bacillus with advantage.

The muscles should be explored by numerous longitudinal incisions, incisions of the muscular sheaths, and the excision of all necrosed tissue, as described on p. 169. The focus of infection, if known, should be excised. The wound should be dressed with the chosen antiseptic solution. The incisions should be kept open by light gauze compresses wet with this solution. No circular bandages which can exert the least compression, and so hinder the escape of the gas, are allowable. Nothing should obstruct the free escape of the gas. Everything should promote it.

If gas gangrene occurs or has already set in, the same free incision should be made, unless this has already been done.

Bacteriologic diagnosis in the early stage is most important. Soon the discoloration of the skin, blebs, and crepitation make the diagnosis positive, but crepitation often appears late rather than early. The x-ray may disclose the bubbles of gas in the tissues. On incision, if the muscular tissue is bloodless, pale, dry, of a brick-red color, gangrene already exists. The best judgment then will be required to decide whether free excision of this gangrenous tissue, with suitable subsequent dressing, or immediate amputation should be done. If the limb is amputated, it should be by the so-called *"guillotine" method*, *i. e., without flaps*. Handley* has an excellent paper with good illustrations on the flapless amputation. The wound should be dressed with the end of the stump entirely uncovered until the infection has been conquered. Then the skin may be drawn down by traction by means of rubber bands or tubing fastened to a splint below and to the stump above by four-ply gauze or calico and glue (*vide* pp. 52-56) or by weights and pulley, and sutured as soon as feasible. The bone may have to be shortened.

* Brit. Med. Jour., August 25, 1917.

AN ANTITOXIN TO PREVENT GAS GANGRENE

One of the most important contributions to the pathology and the treatment of gas gangrene as a result of the war is a series of papers by Carroll G. Bull and Ida W. Pritchett, of the Rockefeller Institute.* It greatly extends, in fact, may be said to revolutionize, our knowledge of the pathology of gas gangrene and its cause. What is still more important and cheering, "it has been possible to produce with it (*i. e.*, with the clear amber filtrate from sterile broth inoculated with a pure culture of the B. Welchii incubated over night at 37° C.) a potent antitoxic serum which will not only neutralize the toxin, so that it produces no lesion, but will inhibit the growth of the bacteria in the body" (Pritchett).

Experiments on animals have led to "the discovery of the conditions under which a highly potent, soluble toxic agent is regularly produced by the bacilli, on which their poisonous or lethal action chiefly, if not wholly, depends."

"This powerful soluble toxin, when injected intravenously, kills animals in a few hours. When injected intramuscularly, it requires more time."

"The cause of death in *Bacillus Welchii* infection is not a blood invasion of the microörganisms and

* See appended bibliography.

not acid intoxication, but an intoxication with definite and very potent poisons produced in the growth of the bacilli in the tissues of the body. . . ."

"The poison or toxin is a complex of an hemolysin and another poisonous body. The latter is the more toxic, since it may bring about death under conditions in which no blood destruction takes place.

"The experiments briefly reported . . . seem to possess considerable importance. They indicate, indeed, that in *Bacillus Welchii* infection in nature the development of the spores into vegetative bacilli may be prevented by a protective inoculation of an antitoxic serum, and also that the vegetative bacilli may be deprived by such a serum of their toxic products, which now appear to be their real offensive instrument. We are confronted, therefore, not only with a new point of view regarding the manner of the pathogenic action of the Welch group of bacilli, but also with a new means of combating their pathogenic effects.

"The experiments presented appear to admit of one interpretation only; namely, that the Welch bacilli, under suitable conditions of growth, produce an active exotoxin, to which their pathogenic effects are ascribable. The toxic product, moreover, acts upon the local tissues and the blood in a manner identical with the action of the cultures. With the toxic product animals may be immunized actively and an immune serum which neutralizes the toxin perfectly and in multiple proportion be secured. The toxic bodies would seem to be at least two in number: one causing blood destruction, hence an hemolysin, and the other acting locally on the tissues and blood-vessels, causing edema and necrosis and probably exerting general toxic action in addition."

These views seem to me to be based on ample experiments and on sound reasoning. Dr. Welch himself has expressed his approval of the conclusions. Some of the antitoxin has already been sent to the surgeons in France, and Dr. Bull is now there to assist in testing the value of the remedy. The results of their tests on the wounded will be awaited with the deepest interest, and it is to be hoped will be conclusively favorable. Doubtless time will also bring improvements in the method as a result of actual use of the antitoxin.

The following are the papers of Bull and Pritchett on their antitoxin against gas gangrene up to March, 1918:

"Toxin and Antitoxin of and Protective Inoculation against B. Welchii," Bull and Pritchett, Jour. Exp. Med., July, 1917.

"Prophylactic and Therapeutic Properties of the Antitoxin for B. Welchii," Bull. Jour. Exp. Med., October, 1917.

"Identity of the Toxins of Different Strains of B. Welchii and Factors Influencing their Production in Vitro," Bull and Pritchett, Jour. Exp. Med., December, 1917.

"Antitoxin for Gaseous Gangrene," Bull, New York Medical Journal, November 3, 1917.

HOSPITAL GANGRENE

Makins, on page 794 of his paper (*loc. cit.*), makes an interesting reference to "Hospital Gangrene," of which, in common with all our surgeons, I saw so much during our Civil War. His description would apply fairly well to those cases, though the rapidly spreading destruction seen in our Civil War cases is not emphasized by Makins. Since then hospital gangrene has entirely disappeared. We do not even know its pathology or its bacteriology. Makins says:

"One form of streptococcus infection deserves special mention as possibly corresponding to the variety of 'classical hospital gangrene' described as the membranous. Cases of this nature have not been common, although sufficiently so to have become familiar. A wound which has previously been apparently progressing favourably becomes covered with a dense grey tough membrane, firmly adherent to the subjacent granulations. In the earliest stage this membrane does not materially differ from the thin layer of coagulated fibrin and included leucocytes which not uncommonly forms in cases of streptococcic infection which, after a time, fail to respond to treatment. The same cessation of free discharge from the wound surface is observed, a condition well described by Colonel Sir Almroth Wright as 'lymph bound.' The membrane then thickens so as to resemble one of the diphtheritic class; in fact, strong suspicion was aroused in the earlier stages of the war that the change was due to a diphtheritic infection. Bacteriological examination has, however, in all cases resulted in the discovery of streptococci alone."

. . . "Amputation is usually followed by a recurrence of the same type of wound surface, and the patient dies in from four days to a week's time after the commencement of the process. No successful method of dealing with this special form of wound infection has been devised."

Our treatment during the Civil War was empirical, but was bacteriologically correct and was very often successful. I would unhesitatingly advise its application to the cases described by Makins. The patient being almost always etherized, the whole wound was cauterized by nitric or nitro-muriatic acid, the acid nitrate of mercury, pure bromin, or the actual cautery. This effectually sterilized the wound. When the slough separated, it was treated as any other fresh wound.

WOUNDS OF THE HEAD

In spite of steel helmets, which have materially reduced their number, wounds of the head are still exceedingly numerous. This is owing to the universal use of trench warfare and on a scale hitherto unknown. While many of these cases find their way into the hospitals, a still larger number die even before they can be collected or sent to a hospital.

"One of the lessons which has been taught us," as Cushing has well pointed out, is that "judgment comes only from special experiences." Two of the best illustrations of the value of experience are seen in the Surgery of the Head and the Surgery of the Jaws: "Only experts can make 50 per cent. of lacerated faces and jaws capable again of army crusts."

Among the communications in the journals dealing with cranial wounds, one of the most judicious, as one would naturally expect, is that by Dr. Harvey Cushing.* His "conclusions" seem to me to be so excellent that I quote them in full:

"There is a fairly universal agreement that almost all cranial wounds produced by projectiles, even

* Military Surgeon, June–July, 1915.

though they appear trivial, require surgical investigation, with the possible exception—(1) of certain of the tangential *longitudinal sinus* injuries, which, according to Sargent and Holmes, have a high degree of spontaneous recoverability, and which, when investigated, present unusual surgical risks; and (2) of certain of the fractures of the base due to perforating wounds, owing to their inaccessibility.

"There is, however, a wide divergence of opinion as to when and where these operations should be performed. It is recognized that cases treated immediately at a field ambulance appear to do well for a time, but are apt to suffer from complications after their evacuation. These complications are often ascribed to the patient's transportation, whereas they are due, in greater probability, to the fact that these early interventions of necessity are hurriedly undertaken and imperfectly executed, and that the wounded must oftentimes be evacuated at about the time when complications from sepsis are likely to occur.

"With the exception of the more serious injuries with extensive hemorrhage, in which surgical measures are practically unavailing, craniocerebral wounds, as a rule, present no immediate urgency, for, as a tissue, the brain is notably tolerant of contusions and infections. Hence a delay of two or three days in forwarding this class of wounded with expedition to a suitable base is preferable to the delay of two or three days in having them recover from the effects of an incomplete procedure before transportation.

"One can rarely tell, from the external appearance of these wounds, how serious a matter the intracranial exploration will prove to be, and if the procedure is abandoned after a trifling crucial incision with a possible trepanation and the removal of a few fragments of bone and clot, followed by a gauze pack, a herniation, fungus, and infection will often ensue.

"Even apparently trivial scalp wounds may in the end require extensive and elaborate operations, which demand a thorough neurologic study, fluoroscopy, or x-ray plates, a carefully planned and deliberate intervention under skilful anesthesia, and the aid of such accessories for the extraction of certain types of missiles as an electromagnet. Accurate closure of the operative wound is desirable, and direct drainage, particularly by gauze, of the area of denuded cortex should be avoided if possible. The success of such a procedure is greatly handicapped by earlier direct enlargements of the original wound."

Especially do I indorse, on general principles, his advice that the only proper hospital to interfere surgically with a cranial wound is one in which facilities in skilled men, both neurologic and surgical, and the best x-ray apparatus, are to be had. At present (April, 1918) some hospitals, much nearer to the trenches than formerly, are thus equipped. An incompletely studied case and an indifferent facility for diagnosis and operation have no place in cranial wounds. The late results of such surgery are lamentable.

Gutter wounds may comminute the skull and produce serious intracranial lesions. As Gamlen and Smith* have pointed out, even through the helmet, and especially at about the temporal crest, though the x-rays show no fracture, though there may be on admission only slight paresis of the face or of an arm, or some aphasia, after two or three days serious cerebral symptoms may arise and require operation. The brain may even be found pulpified. Archibald† confirms this wide-spread destructive action, which may extend to the ventricles and even the optic thalamus. These cases have been often incompletely operated on at busy first-line hospitals and passed on with gauze packing, thus inviting infection.

Archibald, in three active months at the front, did not see a single case of meningitis. He ascribes most of the deaths to "*commotio,*" "that most infernal jostle which the lateral force given off in the passage

* Brit. Jour. Surg., July, 1917.
† Canadian Med. Assoc. Jour., September, 1916.

of a high velocity bullet [or fragment of shell] imparts to the brain."

Decompression operations may relieve increased intracranial pressure. Sargent and Holmes* have used with advantage contralateral decompression. This has the great advantage of being done in clean tissue. If, however, the decompression is done on the same side as the wound, then to protect the brain from the infected scalp flap they recommend that the scalp be widely loosened from the skull, and that one or two pedunculated flaps of pericranium be slid over the brain and carefully sutured in place, prior to the closure of the scalp wound.

In operations on cranial wounds, when possible, access should be had through an independent clean incision, rather than by enlarging the almost certainly infected original wound. Foreign bodies in the brain should be extracted as soon as a complete operation can be done, for in this war practically all such foreign bodies are infected. But the surgeon must use his good judgment and not venture beyond the limits of reasonably legitimate surgery. Sometimes a secondary operation at a much later date will be best. Between the danger of infection and the danger of operation only a large experience and good judg-

* Brit. Med. Jour., March 27 and November 30, 1915.

ment can decide. Occasionally a powerful electromagnet may remove a missile, provided it is of a metal which is amenable to such treatment. The vibrations caused by an intermittent current may aid in loosening the foreign body. The value of the x-ray, especially in the present improved forms, is insisted on (*vide* p. 123 *et seqq.*).

Whether a case can bear immediate transportation is decided largely by the pulse. If it be rapid, the patient should not be forwarded at once. A slow pulse favors the presumption of possible recovery. Such patients, as a rule, will bear transportation lasting even for two or three days. Moreover, an immediate operation at or near the front is not only apt to be an incomplete operation, but is often followed by a great drop in the blood-pressure. A moderate delay is a benefit. Bowlby[*] summarizes the treatment as follows:

"A primary cleansing of the wound. The transmission of the patient as soon as possible to the hospital, where he will convalesce. The taking of x-ray pictures. The excision of the scalp and bone wound. A limited and careful removal of foreign bodies. The covering of the exposed brain. The closure of the wound, with superficial drainage, and a prolonged rest in bed."

[*] Brit. Med. Jour., June 2, 1917.

Archibald* says that by far the best drain [if any is to be used] is Sargent's. It is made of aluminum with wide meshes.

The above views are reinforced also by Makins,† who says:

"Examination of a considerable number of patients some months after their return to England proved much more satisfactory than had been generally expected. It was found that the proportion of patients who die after transference to England is small; later complications, such as cerebral abscess, are comparatively rare, and serious sequelæ, such as insanity and epilepsy, are much less common than had been foretold. In only 15 per cent. of the patients examined, however, had more than one year elapsed from the date of the injury. It also appeared that many patients with foreign bodies deeply lodged in the brain recover, and are scarcely more liable to serious complications than men in whom the brain has been merely exposed and lacerated. These conclusions are obviously tentative, but as far as they go appear hopeful."

Sargent (in Bowlby's paper), from a very large experience, confirms the same:

"The very large experience gained of gunshot wounds of the head has led to a considerable degree

* Canad. Med. Assoc. Jour., September, 1916.
† Brit. Med. Jour., June 16, 1917.

of modification in their treatment. Immediate routine operation, often incomplete, and, in the absence of full neurological information and x-ray examination, sometimes unnecessary and even misdirected, is no longer widely practised. It has long since been made abundantly clear that early evacuation of operated cases is often followed by disaster. As it is impossible to operate upon these cases and to retain them at the clearing stations for a period which renders transportation safe, more especially during times of great military activity, the practice now generally adopted is to transfer them without operation as soon as possible to hospitals further down the line. It has been made quite clear that surgical intervention is rarely required for the relief of cerebral symptoms, whether general or focal. Its chief aim is the prevention of intradural infection. On this conception all cases of gunshot wounds of the head fall into one of two categories, according to whether the dura mater has or has not been penetrated. Non-penetrating wounds have a low rate of mortality, whether operated upon or not, provided that the surgeon respects the integrity of the dura mater.

"It is customary, therefore, to do in these cases only as much as may seem advisable to ensure speedy healing, such as excision of the edges of the wound, removal where necessary of bony fragments, and partial or complete closure of the gap in the scalp either by suture or by some form of plastic operation."

Penetrating wounds should be treated conservatively, as indicated by Bowlby.

As to retained missiles, Sargent says:

"Removal of bullets, even when the wounds have healed and the risk of septic infection thereby is largely diminished, must be, even in skilled hands, attended by an amount of damage which, in most cases, would have more serious neurological consequences than could the presence of an aseptic bullet.

"Primary removal of a deeply seated missile carries with it the additional risk of septic infection. For these reasons the usual practice is to leave alone such missiles."

For many years I have formulated the following rule, taught it to my numerous classes, and have always found it satisfactory. "If the surgeon, by seeking to extract a missile retained in the brain, will do more harm than the missile, do not operate" —and vice versa. Later, epilepsy may develop. In this case, except for the removal of a foreign body or an indriven fragment of bone,—always to be determined by the x-ray examination,—no operation should be done. Even if such foreign bodies are accurately located, they may be so deeply embedded as to make it inadvisable to attempt to remove them.

Moreover, no one should decide upon operation after only one or two attacks, even of Jacksonian epilepsy. If, however, they recur more often, then a carefully planned operation may be advised.

Holmes and Sargent,* after a study of over 70 cases, have described "The Longitudinal Sinus Syndrome." The paper cannot well be summarized, but their conclusions as to treatment are concise and reasonable. As a rule, do not operate. If operation be done, secure ample access to control the almost certain serious hemorrhage which can often be controlled by the implantation of raw muscle often to be obtained from the flap itself (Horsley).

Makins rightly calls attention to a valuable paper by Lister and Gordon Holmes entitled "Disturbances of Vision from Cerebral Lesions, with Especial Reference to the Cerebral Representation of the Macula."† It is fully illustrated and is a most important contribution both to cerebral localization and to the physiology of vision. It is particularly creditable that men so constantly overworked should persistently continue their scientific researches.

* "Injuries of the Superior Longitudinal Sinus," Jour. Royal Army Med. Corps, 1915, xxv, p. 56.

† Proc. Roy. Soc. Med., 1916, ix, Section on Ophthalmology, p. 57.

I cannot do better than conclude this section with a résumé of Cushing's latest paper.*

He was the chief of one of three hospitals devoted to injuries of the head. Of the 225 cases in his own hospital, 6 died without operation. The remaining 219 cases were all operated on. In 133 the dura was penetrated. Of these 133 there were—

	OPERATIONS	DEATHS	PERCENTAGE OF MORTALITY
In the first month	44	24	54.5
In the second month	44	18	40.9
In the third month	45	13	28.8

That is, the mortality was almost cut in half. His conviction is that a mortality rate of only 25 per cent. is attainable.

It is noteworthy that so experienced and able a surgeon as Cushing frankly states that with enlarging experience his skill became greater, and, as shown above, his mortality percentages were practically cut in half. The rest of us may well take courage that with study and experience we too may do as well.

The operative procedure he evolved may be summarized from his paper thus:

* Brit. Med. Jour., February 23, 1918.

"1. The *removal en bloc* rather than piecemeal of the *area of cranial penetration.*

"2. *The detection of the indriven bony fragments by catheter palpation of the track* rather than by the exploring finger.

"3. The *suction method of removal of the disorganized brain*" tissue, similar in effect to the excision of the devitalized tissue in other wounds.

"4. *The use of dichloramin-T in oils as an antiseptic.*" Prior to operation he insists on certain important points.

(a) The organization of an *operating team* as "a prime consideration. Every such team should be provided with an extra wooden operating table,—if possible with two,"—so that the preoperative steps (neurologic examination, x-ray, shaving of scalp and giving the anesthetic) of the succeeding case can go on coincidentally with the operation and so no time be lost—and time is precious there, especially as hardly more than eight serious cases can be operated on in the working day. "An extra table is almost as valuable as an extra medical officer."

(b) A thorough *neurologic examination* should be made and *recorded* for later reference in order to determine whether the symptoms have changed for better or for worse, and whether new symptoms have appeared.

(c) Good *x-ray pictures* should be taken.

(d) The *entire* scalp should be *shaved*. "Shaving of the scalp is an art, requires a good barber, and is indispensable." He rejects the clippers because "they leave short hairs difficult to remove." Instead of that, a "short hair cut," before going into battle, is desirable. For the wounded he advises a warm soap poultice at the field ambulance, as it is a good preventive of infection, and makes the operative preparation of the scalp—"no easy task when an uncropped head of hair has become caked with blood and mud—less arduous." Sponging with alcohol and bichlorid he prefers to iodin or picric acid.

(e) An hour before operation ⅓ grain of *omnopon* is given and repeated if necessary. Fifteen to twenty minutes before operation the scalp is infiltrated in the lines of the incision with a 1 per cent. solution of *novocain and adrenalin* (15 drops to 30 c.c.) injected into the subaponeurotic layer. He far prefers local anesthesia to general anesthesia, and gives several excellent reasons for his preference. A few exceptional cases may require general anesthesia.

(f) In a few cases the usual flap with the wound in its center may be used, but much more frequently a *tripod* or a "three-legged Isle of Man" incision is the best (Figs. 47 and 48). The flaps should be "undermined" if there is tension when they are sutured. He sutures the galea capitis with fine black silk,

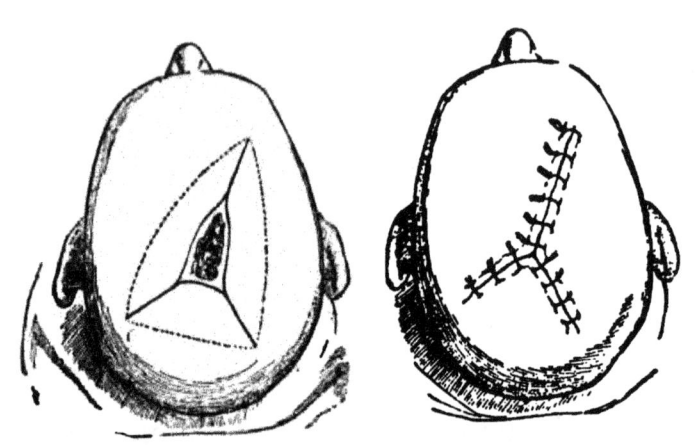

Fig. 47.—Tripod incision for small irregular wound of vault. Dotted lines indicate area of reflection of flaps (Cushing, in British Medical Journal).

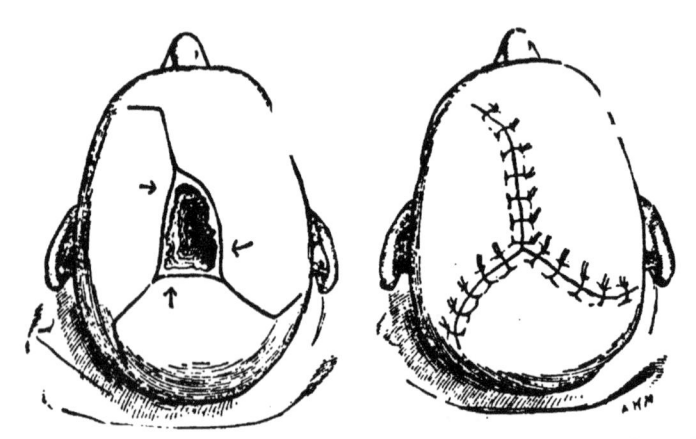

Fig. 48.—Three-legged (Isle of Man) incisions for larger wound of cranial vault (Cushing, in British Medical Journal).

the rest of the scalp with the same, and removes the sutures in the scalp on the second day. He eschews silkworm gut entirely and for good reasons.

(g) For opening the skull he "encircles the area of depressed bone with a number of small" openings made by a perforator and burr and connects them by the Montenovesi cranial forceps (Fig. 49), the merits of which he states, and tilts the disc of bone out in one piece (Fig. 50). This has several advantages, the most important being that in case of severe hemorrhage, especially if a sinus is wounded, there is

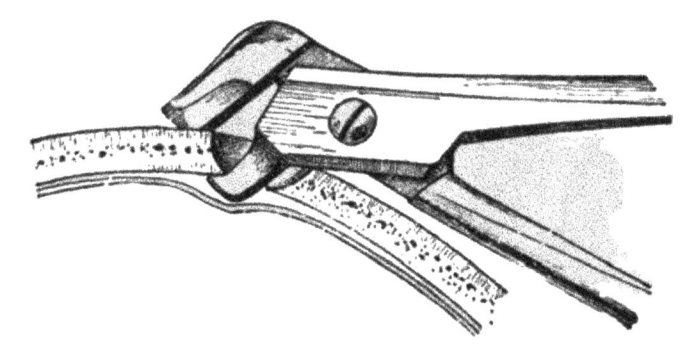

Fig. 49.—Montenovesi linear cutting forceps to follow burr (Cushing, in British Medical Journal).

ample "elbow room" to deal with it. The hemorrhage can often be sealed by a muscle graft.

(h) *The thorough cleaning of the track of the missile is "the most important step of the operation,"* for it means the removal of the devitalized tissue lining the track and the indriven fragments of bone. As we have seen in other wounds, such tissue is the best possible soil for cultivation of bacteria and especially of the most dangerous anaërobes of tetanus and gas gangrene. Colonel Gray has suggested—another advantage of local anesthesia—that the patient could cough, by which clots and cerebral débris are often expelled.

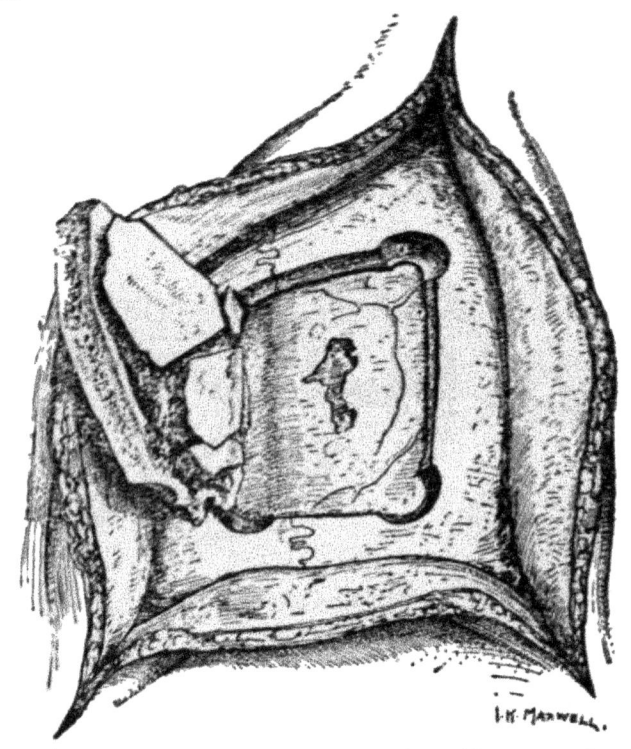

Fig. 50.—Showing the turning back from the mid-vertex of an area of depressed fracture (actual specimen), disclosing a dural laceration with tear to the margin of the sinus (Cushing, in British Medical Journal).

Cushing relies on a *soft-rubber catheter* "as a means of determining the exact direction taken by the missile, whether metallic, bone fragments, or both, with great satisfaction (Fig. 51).

"By attaching to the end of the catheter a Carrel-

WOUNDS OF THE HEAD

Gentile glass syringe with its rubber bulb (Fig. 52) it is possible to suck up into its lumen the softened brain, which can then be expelled from the catheter as paste is expressed from the orifice of a tube. The

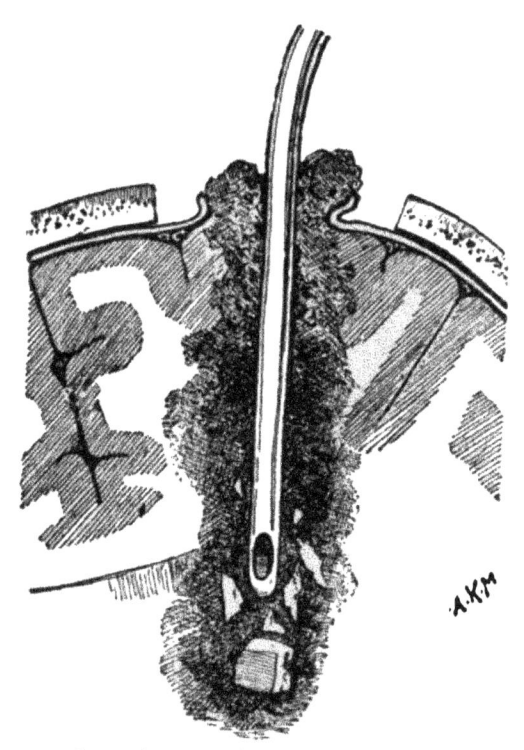

Fig. 51.—Diagram to show the insertion of a catheter in the track of a penetrating missile (Cushing, in British Medical Journal).

process should be repeated until the cavity is rendered as free as possible of all the softened and infiltrated brain. It will be found that the adjoining normal cerebral tissue, unaffected by the original contusion, will not be drawn into the tube by the degree of suction which can be applied by the average rubber bulb.

"Fragments of bone can be felt by the catheter and removed from the track by delicate duck-billed forceps."

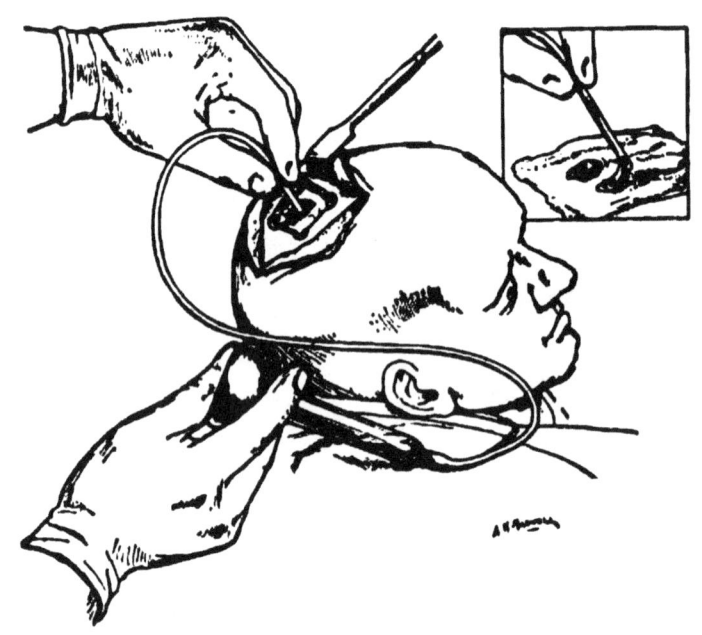

Fig. 52.—Sketch illustrating the method of suction of the track of a penetrating wound (Cushing, in British Medical Journal).

In 25 cases the ventricles have been opened. "Many such cases have made good recoveries."

In 1890, at the International Medical Congress in Berlin, I presented a long paper on the "Surgery of the Lateral Ventricles." It was an elaborate study of all the recorded ventricular cases from Ambroise Paré's time, including my own successful cases. I can, therefore, fully confirm Cushing's statement.*

(*i*) The dura should only be opened—and with stringent precautions against infection—in case of serious loss of function or if the tense dura evidently overlies a clot or a severely contused area. After proper treatment the dura is sutured with fine black silk in curved French needles [not with heavy needles with cutting edges and coarse sutures].

"If the surgeon has any doubts of his technic or of the cleanliness of the wound," he should not open the dura.

(*k*) As to removal of missiles, each individual case must be decided upon its own merits. The rule I (K.) have quoted on page 187 I think will serve. Of

* The later history of this paper is interesting. I had spent upon it all the leisure time at my disposal for nearly a year and devoted to it a week in the Surgeon General's Library in Washington. Immediately after reading it I personally placed the MS. (some 100 pages of typewritten MS.) in the hands of the Secretary of the Surgical Section, the late Prof. Sonnenburg. A year later Professor von Bergmann, President of the Section, cabled me for the MS. I cabled him the facts. He replied that the MS. had been lost! Unfortunately I had no carbon copy! I also wrote to Sonnenburg. The latter neither answered my letter nor explained nor apologized for the asserted loss. Only a brief "Referat" therefore appears in the Transactions of the Congress.

course, superficially lodged missiles should always be removed. Deep-seated ones may be removed in some suitable cases by a powerful magnet. Cushing describes his procedure. The foreign body is reached by means of a French wire nail. He has thus removed 11 foreign bodies.

(*l*) For later treatment he has used dichloramin-T with satisfaction.

The entire article should be read and "inwardly digested." Also the editorial in the same issue of the Journal.

Following immediately after Cushing's paper is one by Rayner and Barclay, describing a most ingenious instrument and method by which they extracted a deep-lying foreign body with great benefit to the patient.

WOUNDS OF THE CHEST

The *missiles* are chiefly bullets or fragments of shell. The former in many cases may almost be said to be innocuous as compared with the wounds caused by fragments of shells. A bullet rather rarely carries in pieces of clothing or other foreign body, but it may fracture one or two ribs and drive fragments of bone into the lung itself as secondary missiles. Occasionally the splinter may be indriven, but remain hinged to the rib and thus wound the lung at every inspiration.

A fragment of shell will generally carry in pieces of infected clothing or dirty skin. In this case infection—even by the fragment of shell alone—is practically certain and most dangerous. (*Cf.* p. 64 and Fig. 23.)

The wound may be only a *penetrating* wound. The bullet or a piece of shell then is retained as a foreign body. If the foreign body is large, it must be removed; if small, it will often, possibly even generally, do less harm if allowed to remain than to remove it, unless it is doing or sure to do harm.

Gask and Wilkinson* define a "large" foreign body as measuring an inch by half an inch. A bullet is usually classed as "small." An x-ray picture should always be made in order to locate such a foreign body and judge of its character, size, and surroundings.

If it be a *perforating* wound, the missile has escaped and we have only to deal with the damage it has done in transit.

The most dangerous wound is one in which a large portion of the chest-wall has been "blown away," leaving an "open chest," *i. e.*, a large hole in the chest-wall, exposing the lung.

The phenomena in wounds of the thorax, in addition to shock, which, especially in an "open chest" wound, is almost sure to be severe, are:

1. Dyspnea.—The degree of the dyspnea depends largely on the size of the opening. If it be only the small wound of entrance of a bullet, there may be but little. If there is a large opening into the chest, the dyspnea will be severe (traumatopnea), the patient gasping for breath. This is due partly to the collapse of the exposed lung and partly or even chiefly by the inability not only of the lung on the wounded side to expand, but because the opposite lung inspires the air with difficulty. When an attempt at

* Brit. Med. Jour., December 15, 1917.

inspiration is made, the air is drawn into the chest through the wide opening of the wound with far greater ease than through the narrower air-passages. Hence the imperative need of closing this gaping wound as quickly as possible. The moment this is accomplished the patient finds great relief from his air-hunger.

2. Hemorrhage.—The hemorrhage from the intercostal arteries may be considerable, but that from the lung itself is usually far more important. If one of the large pulmonary vessels is divided, the patient may easily die in a very short time on the field itself, not living long enough to reach even the first-aid station.

Ordinarily, therefore, those actually treated suffer chiefly from hemorrhage from the medium-sized pulmonary vessels. Death from this cause usually occurs in from twenty-four to forty-eight hours. In these cases, as pointed out by Moynihan (American Addresses on War Surgery, Saunders, 1917, p. 125), "both in the French and English armies precocious operative means are being adopted . . . with a degree of success that encourages a wide adoption of this practice."

3. Hemothorax is very frequent. An *x*-ray picture will show the shadow of the hemothorax. If

the amount is such as to cause serious dyspnea, early aspiration should be done, but slowly—Rees and Hughes and also Rudolf say not over one ounce a minute. If the amount of accumulated blood is moderate (Elliott says not over 30 ounces), and *if it is sterile*, nature will absorb it with less danger than the surgeon can remove it by operation.

The question of the condition of the accumulated blood is vital. *If sterile*, it may be left alone for a week or more and then aspirated if it is not being absorbed. If, on the other hand, it is *infected*, then, unless other conditions forbid, the earlier it is removed the better. Whether sterile or infected can best be decided by an exploratory aspiration to obtain a "sample" of the fluid by a hypodermic needle with a long enough needle to insure reaching through the chest-wall and a possibly thickened pleura. Moynihan (*loc. cit.*) quotes Henry's statement that, out of 500 tappings, 195 showed infection, of which 87 were by anaërobic organisms. But he warns the surgeon that puncture in the upper, fluid portion of the hemothorax may show no organisms, while one made lower down, into the more solid fibrinous clot, may give positive results. The lesson is clear: *two* diagnostic punctures should be made at different levels.

If infection is shown, then immediate thoracotomy

is indicated unless there be weighty reasons to the contrary (*vide infra*).

The opposite lung—as this war has shown, according to Moynihan—is frequently, and in severe cases probably always injured. Disseminated hemorrhages beneath the pleura or in the pulmonary substance take place, and in later stages areas of bronchopneumonia are found.

Treatment.—This has in part been indicated already. First and foremost, as in fractures, as *complete physical immobility* as is possible. Absolute rest in bed, speaking only when it is imperative, making no effort to aid the nurse or orderly when the bladder or bowels are emptied or when being fed. Even turning the patient on his side to dress his wound must be avoided if possible, as death has followed such a maneuver. The patient must *not* be evacuated further down the line, but be kept in the station where he has been treated, which should be at the "dressing station" or "field hospital," according to military conditions.

If the case is one of *perforation* of a bullet or a shrapnel ball, the missile escaping, and there be no evidence of serious hemorrhage or other complication, the skin should be fully disinfected, both wounds excised, and a simple protective dressing applied, securely kept in place by adhesive plaster and bandages.

If the ball or bullet has *lodged* and the x-ray shows that it may not cause later mischief, the case may also be treated conservatively.

If the missile is a fragment of shell, it will almost certainly cause infection, and, as a rule, should be removed. Other wounds should be taken into account in reaching a final decision.

For *hemorrhage*, if progressive and threatening during the first day or two,—after that it rarely occurs,—a thoracotomy exposing the lung is requisite. The hemorrhage should be checked not by plugging but by catgut suture, which is very effective and speedy. If any "large" foreign body is present, it should be removed by incision of the lung tissue if it is embedded in the lung. The incision should be sutured at once. Splinters of bone, loose, embedded in the lung, or indriven and connected with the chest-wall, should be removed; the pleura carefully but quickly cleansed of blood and any other foreign body, and the wound closed.

If the case is one of "open thorax," the chief indication is to close the opening in the chest-wall as quickly as possible consistent with other conditions. If pleura can be approximated to pleura, this should be done, followed by muscle to muscle and skin to skin. Very likely the first will be impossible; in that case the gap must be filled with muscle, or if this is wanting, then by skin, a flap or flaps being utilized if necessary. Unless closure is effected, infection is certain. Grégoire in 17 cases was successful in 16 (Moynihan).

If the hemothorax has become infected—*i. e.*, if it has become a case of "empyema," one of two courses is open, according to the needs of the case. If it is a simple empyema, the old method in civil practice has usually been to remove a small piece of rib and insert a drainage-tube. But weeks and even months often passed before healing took place, if it ever did heal. Tuffier, as noted by Moynihan, has profoundly modified the treatment of such cases. Instead of inserting one large drainage-tube, Tuffier advises that the Carrel-Dakin treatment be immediately instituted, viz., several small tubes threaded on wire are placed in different positions in the cavity. An *x*-ray picture will show if they have been properly located. "A little loose gauze is packed into the wound and a safety tube for drainage of excess fluid is placed in one angle of the incision. Dakin's fluid is then instilled in the usual manner. At the end of ten days all discharge has ceased (there is rarely more than an extremely small quantity after the first two days) the tubes are then removed and the wound closed."

If, on the other hand, a more extensive operation has to be done for breaking up adhesions and for the removal of foreign bodies, as well as evacuating the purulent fluid, then the more serious operation well described by Moynihan must be undertaken.

He has his patient lying on his back with his arms at his sides. An incision five to six inches long is made along the fourth rib. The fibers of the great pectoral are separated—those of the lesser are separated from the rib. Hemostasis should be complete. The periosteum is now divided along the middle of the rib for five inches and stripped off from the rib. Five inches of the rib may be resected or divided anteriorly and fractured, but not detached posteriorly, and replaced when the operation is over. Care must be taken not to wound the pleura, as it must be utilized in closing the wound. It should be separated from the two adjacent ribs above and below, and incised horizontally. The ribs are then retracted up and down and the whole hand is inserted. Adhesions are to be gently torn as in the abdomen. The collapsed lung now will lie free in the pleural cavity and can be delivered much as a kidney can be by a little "coaxing." It is to be surrounded by cloths wrung out of warm normal saline solution. A foreign body, bullet, shell fragment, splinter of bone, etc., can then easily be felt and removed through an incision which is immediately sutured by catgut. Deep stitches are used if necessary.

The lung is then returned, the pleural cavity carefully cleaned. Moynihan advises wiping "a gauze swab wet with ether over the visceral pleura and any adhesions which may have been separated." Then the pleura is sutured—often a difficult procedure—the muscles and skin carefully sutured in layers, and the ether and air withdrawn from the pleural cavity by a needle. "The lung then rapidly expands and faint breath-sounds are heard at once," and with great joy, I venture to add.

One other serious form of injury of the chest is called the "Stove-in Chest" by Lockwood and Nixon.* In these cases there may be even no external wound, yet the bony framework may have been crushed in and fractured. The soft parts may be lacerated and the ribs be comminuted, resulting in sharp bony spicules. The pleura also may be badly torn. The lungs and the heart may also be injured. Shock is, of course, very severe. Until they operated on these stove-in cases practically every one died.

* Brit. Med. Jour., January 26, 1918.

Lockwood and Nixon advise against the use of ether or chloroform in wounds of the chest.

A large number of thoracic wounds pierce the diaphragm, and therefore involve also the abdominal cavity. Sometimes the missiles may enter the abdomen first and reach the chest last. In every case in which the diaphragm has been injured Lockwood and Nixon strongly advise operation. At first they repaired the diaphragmatic wound from the abdomen, but later through the thorax. The viscera of the abdomen may be wounded or may escape injury. The treatment of these visceral injuries is practically the same as if the chest had not suffered injury as well. Such cases of combined injuries are exceedingly dangerous and demand immediate attention and the best balanced judgment.

Mortality.—Pierre Duval (*vide* Moynihan, *loc. cit.*, p. 117) has collected 3455 cases, with a mortality of 688—about 20 per cent. He, however, arrived at a quite different result when he analyzed the mortality in different stations from the firing line to the base hospitals. At the first-aid post the mortality is about 25 per cent., so that of 100 patients, 75 will be evacuated down the line. At the "ambulance"— *i. e.*, an early hospital—20 per cent. more will die, leaving 60 to be evacuated to the base hospitals.

There 10 per cent. more will die, leaving only 54 who finally recover. These estimates do not include those who die on the field and never reach even the first-aid station. Were these included, the mortality of *all* wounds of the chest would be considerably above one-half.

Depage at La Panne in 320 cases states that the mortality in the first twenty-four hours was 9.4, chiefly from hemorrhage. The mortality of the remainder was 10 per cent., chiefly from sepsis. The mortality of the whole series—those who died on the field, of course, were not included—was 18.4 per cent., a far more favorable result than that given by Duval. In either case the death-rate is very high. Our best efforts are needed to reduce this serious loss.

WOUNDS OF THE JOINTS

The military surgery of joints is, *par excellence*, that of the knee. Bowlby's remarks on these injuries* are well worth quoting in part:

"A great change for the better has taken place in the results obtained in the treatment of wounded joints. . . .

"Experience was chiefly gained on the knee-joint, for it is the joint most frequently hit, most easy of inspection, and its infection is followed by disastrous consequences more often than in the case of other articulations. . . .

"The first improvement was the abandonment of the intra-articular drains. The next was the excision of the wound, the removal of any foreign body, the flushing of the joint, and in some cases the closure of the capsule and the insertion of a superficial drain. . . .

"The next step was perhaps a bold one. As soon as possible after the receipt of the injury—that is, in the casualty clearing station—the wound was excised, the joint opened, cleaned, and irrigated, and then the whole wound in the synovial sac and the

* Brit. Med. Jour., June 2, 1917.

superficial tissues was tightly closed. It was certainly astonishing how seldom infection followed such treatment, even when fragments of shell or pieces of clothing had been removed from the joint; but for its success it is essential that the incisions around the wound edges should be carried quite clear of all infected tissue, and that the strictest asepsis is assured.

"Now, every knee-joint with such a wound is given the chance of healing by first intention, although the closure of the joint defect may entail the performance of a plastic operation to provide an adequate cover with a flap of synovial membrane or skin. Even if some infection does follow the closure of the joint, it is well not to be in too great hurry to lay the articulation open, for a certain number of such joints do settle down and provide a better limb than if submitted to more active treatment.

"When the joint wound is complicated with fracture of bone, it may still be possible in some cases to close it with success. In cases of compound fracture of the patella with loss of substance, partial or complete removal of the fragments, and the provision of a skin-flap, will often be followed by primary healing.

"When the tibia or femur is involved the case becomes more serious. Of the two fractures, that of the tibia is the most to be feared."

The "bold step" of primary closure of the joint is clearly justified by the following statistics from a table including 845 cases of injury to the knee-joint in Barling's hospital in Rouen.* The part which I reproduce is very impressive. The contrast as to re-operation between the cases of excision and *closure*, and excision and *packing*, is most instructive.

1. Total cases of injury to knee operated on.............................. 845
2. With bone injury................. 438
3. Without bone injury.............. 407
4. Wound excised and closed......... 322
5. Cases with wounds excised and *closed* requiring further operation........ 82 = 25.5 per cent.
6. Wound excised and packed......... 336
7. Cases with wounds excised and *packed* requiring further operation........ 128 = 38.4 per cent.

Acquaintance with the later literature of gunshot wounds of the joints confirms the opinion above expressed and shows practical unanimity of opinion. When the wound is a simple perforating wound by bullet or shrapnel ball, free excision of the wound and immediate closure give remarkable results. These consist not only of healing of the wound and saving both life and limb, but in giving the patient a *good movable joint* in a notable percentage of cases.

If drainage-tubes are used, one finds in most of the articles the now classic phrase, insert them "down to but not in to the joint."

* Barling, Brit. Med. Jour., September 1, 1917.

The very first indication for treatment is again as perfect *immobilization* as possible and also again best by the Thomas splint.

If the *projectile has lodged.* Before any treatment is decided upon, every wound of a joint should be "*x*-rayed" for the double purpose of determining— (1) if the bones have been injured, and, if so, the nature and extent of the injury, and (2) of determining whether there is any foreign body lodged in or near the joint.

A bullet or a shrapnel ball, if superficial and easily reached, should be removed. This is best done by a new clean incision rather than through the track of the wound. If, however, it is embedded in the cancellous extremity of one of the bones and is *not* projecting into the joint, it may usually be left undisturbed until a much later period, when all danger of sepsis has passed. Even then, if not causing any damage, it may be disregarded. In 1862 I assisted Professor S. D. Gross in removing a leaden bullet from the leg of a French soldier who had received a flesh wound at the battle of the Borodino in Napoleon's Russian campaign. It had remained encapsulated in the soft parts (not in the bone) for fifty years, had caused the gradual formation of a cup of bony tissue, which finally resulted in a superficial abscess. Similar encapsulation in cancellous bone tissue also easily takes place. If, however, the foreign body protrudes into the joint cavity, and especially if it is a piece of shell, and more especially if it is a fragment of clothing and is not removed, it will certainly give rise to a most dangerous infection of the joint.

Prevention of a serious arthritis should be the aim of the surgeon. The whole leg for say six or eight inches above and below the joint should be thoroughly disinfected. The skin surrounding the aperture and the track of the wound should then be carefully excised all in one piece. Some surgeons first disinfect the track of the wound by the actual cautery, so as to prevent infection during excision. The incision should always afford easy access, both by sight and touch, to the foreign body in the joint. Blood-clot and any small splinters of bone should be gently removed and the synovial membrane closed except at one place, where a drainage-tube, extending "down to but not in to the joint," may be placed for say twenty-four hours or a day or two longer if necessary. When the synovial membrane cannot be closed, Gray[*] makes the excellent suggestion that the large suprapatellar pouch of the synovial mem-

[*] Brit. Med. Jour., September 1, 1917.

brane be loosened by the finger or the curved scissors from its upper and anterior connections and pulled down. Then apply a sterile dressing and always a splint for immobility. "The surgeon who exhibits the greatest care in technique, especially when removing foreign bodies and infected tissue, whether of the soft parts or the bone," he rightly says, "gets the best results." This means changing of gloves, instruments, towels, etc., one or more times during the operation.

A moderate post-operative reaction will very probably follow, but unless serious infection has occurred, recovery with a mobile joint will follow in a large number of cases.

If, however, an arthritis sets in, with distention of the joint by fluid, and the temperature and pulse rise, then an immediate bacteriologic examination will show the degree of danger. The ordinary pyogenic bacteria will cause an arthritis which may subside in a short time. If the streptococcus is found, it always creates a grave—and it may be a very grave—situation which demands immediate action. So, too, if the infection is caused by the ordinary pyogenic bacteria and does not quickly subside, the same course must be pursued.

The joint should be opened by long incisions on

both sides of the joint, or it may be necessary to make a large anterior flap by a U incision, with division of the ligamentum patellæ. Campbell and Woolfenden,[*] Moynihan,[†] Barling,[‡] and others then advocate the immediate institution of the Carrel-Dakin method of progressive sterilization. When the joint has become "clinically sterile," then the wound is closed. Not a few of these most threatening cases recover with a movable joint!

If, however, the case goes from bad to worse, resection of the joint or amputation may be absolutely necessary.

Resection of joints may be advisable in some cases, but the grave warning of Sir Robert Jones should be heeded (*vide* pp. 56–58). "The functional results," as seen in the many cases finally seeking treatment in the 16 orthopedic centers in England, he says, "are very bad. Flail knees, flail elbows, flail shoulders— many of them suppurating—are constantly in evidence." It is evident, therefore, that the surgeon should be extremely cautious in deciding upon an excision, and if it be done, that the amount of bone removed should be the minimum that is necessary.

[*] Lancet, August 11, 1917.
[†] American Address, p. 80.
[‡] *Loc. cit.*

Flail joints in the arm are bad enough, but in the leg they are possibly worse.

When ankylosis is the object in view, Sir Robert Jones also lays down certain principles as to the position of the limb, which are of great practical importance.

"If the *shoulder* is excised, the arm should be placed in an abducted position at an angle of about 50 degrees. The elbow should be slightly in front of the coronal plane of the body, so that when it is at a right angle and the forearm is supinated, the palm of the hand is toward the face . . .

"Excision of the *elbow*, with complete removal of the condyles and the olecranon, generally leads to flail elbow—a most useless elbow to a working-man. On the other hand, an elbow ankylosed firmly at nearly a right angle is very serviceable . . . The worst cases . . . are those which have been kept straight with the hand pronated." He advises 70 degrees flexion from full extension, the forearm nearly two-thirds supinated."

"The *wrist* should be in dorsi-flexion; the *hips* in slight abduction and external rotation with full extension; the *knee* in full extension; the *ankle* at a right angle and very slightly varoid."

In many cases there is *serious injury to the bone or*

bones—extensive fissured fractures or the destruction of a considerable portion of the articular end of one or both bones. The x-ray picture will reveal the conditions. The Army Medical Museum in Washington has a large collection of such injuries gathered during the Civil War, revealing slight damage in some cases, but most extensive injuries in the majority.

After the battle of Antietam I sent to this museum, from the hospitals in Frederick, Maryland, a large number of postmortem specimens of such wounds of the knee-joint—I think there were twenty, every one of which, with our then septic methods, should have been amputated! Our treatment of such wounds was by drainage and the "antiphlogistic" regimen! How archaic even the very name now sounds, carrying us back to the days before Priestley. Similar cases today would doubtless result in a recovery rate of well over 50 per cent., and not a few of them with movable joints!

The *treatment* should be conservative or radical, according to the conditions found.

In a fair proportion of these cases the x-ray picture may enable us to decide at once whether *amputation* is needful, or whether conservative methods are justifiable. If in doubt, the joint should be freely opened as already indicated, and widely enough to see clearly the existing conditions. If the popliteal vessels have been wounded, amputation should be done at once, without even delaying for the x-rays.

If these vessels are intact, then the method described on pp. 215-16 with the Carrel-Dakin treatment may hold out hope—a hope also not uncommonly realized.

Sir Berkeley Moynihan[*] gives testimony to the "remarkable degree of restoration that had been obtained" in some cases of severe infection of the knee by the use of Mr. Morison's "Bipp." (*Vide ante*, pp. 118 *et seqq.*)

[*] *Loc. cit.*, p. 82.

ABDOMINAL WOUNDS

The experience of the Boer War led us toward abstention in abdominal wounds unless there was suspected hemorrhage or fair evidence of visceral lesion. This was due to the small jacketed bullet, which not seldom traversed the abdominal cavity without wounding any viscus. Wallace states that only 207 abdominal cases were reported in that war, whereas* he reports 1200 cases and 965 operations!

In the present war, especially of late, the bomb, grenade, and high explosive shell have changed all this. Rarely, in case of penetration, do the viscera escape. Hence the burden of proof has been shifted. Abdominal section is now the rule unless there is good reason to believe that *no* hollow viscus at least has been wounded. The "Observation Ward" (see p. 20) will be especially useful in "doubtful" abdominal cases.

After having done 500 emergency operations, Walters, Robinson, Jordan, and Banksmith† add

* Brit. Jour. Surg., iv, p. 679.
† Lancet, February 10, 1917.

the weight of so large an experience in favor of early operation. *Every hour* diminishes such a patient's chances. But even such cases may sometimes benefit by a delay of one or two hours for warmth and rest. Of their 500 operations, 245 recovered and 255 died—a recovery rate of 49 per cent.

Wallace, and Hughes and Rees* give encouraging statistics as to operative interference in abdominal wounds, showing a reduction in mortality of some 10 per cent. at the front. The importance of the earliest possible operation is emphasized especially by the figures of the last two surgeons. Patients operated on within the first six hours (43 in number) showed a recovery percentage of 62.8 per cent. In those operated on between six and twelve hours (33 cases) this had fallen to 36.3 per cent. In operations done between twelve and sixteen hours (18 cases) it had fallen to 16.6 per cent. After over twenty-four hours (11 cases) the recovery rate rose to 45.4 per cent. This can be readily accounted for on the ground that the more seriously wounded had already succumbed.

In *intestinal* cases Bowlby (note to the paper by Walters and colleagues, Lancet, February 10, 1917, p. 207) lays stress on *not operating if the case is seen*

* Lancet, April 28, 1917.

more than thirty-six hours after the wound was received. Out of "many hundreds" of such operations he knows of "only three or four recoveries!" He also strongly advises against operating on patients wounded in the region of the liver by a through-and-through wound. He has seen more harm than good from such operations. A serious wound of the liver is usually fatal; if not serious, hemorrhage has probably ceased and the patient can wait.

One sentence I approve of, though I suspect it may meet with dissent. "Exploration by the finger and probe should be done whenever possible." In these days it is not necessary to add "by the *carefully disinfected* finger and probe," for that goes without saying. No finger or probe that has not been carefully disinfected should ever touch any wound. But I believe that, used with this precaution, they give us much reliable information which cannot be obtained otherwise.

In judging of the course of the missile it should be remembered that the recumbent posture in which we examine the patient is rarely his posture when he was wounded. It is one of the oldest rules of military surgery to put the patient in the position in which he was wounded. In cases of a serious wound preventing the patient from leaving his bed, we can put an orderly in the position required, and by marking the wound of entrance and exit on his skin, can judge of the course of the missile—a practice we often followed during the Civil War.

A good illustration of how a hospital may be suddenly flooded with operative cases is given by Lockwood and his colleagues.* After being rushed with the wounded from four days of continuous active fighting, suddenly in one night, between 9 and 12 o'clock, 96 operative cases—one every two minutes—were received. Of these, 36 were abdominal cases, and of these, 32 were operated on. One significant statement is that the surgeon "was usually obliged to operate alone." This is much less likely now.

Not uncommonly the missile reaches the abdomen through the back and the buttock, instead of from the front. Such wounds are apt to be *very* dangerous from hemorrhage, sepsis, or retroperitoneal cellulitis.

It is very often a question whether operation should be done at once after the patient has been transported over a rough road, and, it may well be, is in marked shock and, in the cold weather, chilled through. Of course, if there is evident hemorrhage, or a strong suspicion of it, immediate operation *must*

* Lockwood, McGill, Kennedy, MacFie, and Charles: Brit. Med. Jour., March 10, 1917.

be done. The usual restoratives, and if possible the measures advocated by Porter and Cannon and his colleagues (*vide* p. 14, *et seqq.*), may be resorted to if the patient's condition requires them. Lockwood and his colleagues base their decision chiefly on the pulse. If this is above 120 beats, operation should be deferred for a reasonable time for reaction to set in.

Walters and his colleagues, and Webb and Milligan,* like Lockwood, point out the value of the pulse as a guide as to operating or not. Their chart shows the relation of the pulse and the mortality. A pulse of 85 to 110 will give the average result of mortality; below 85 the prognosis is good; above 110, it is bad.

The incision should not include the wound of entrance nor cross the track of the wound, as infection may readily spread widely from such an incision. The position of the wound is of great value, especially if both the wounds of entrance and exit are present. The same is true if the lodged bullet is found. Escape of the contents of the stomach, intestine, gall-bladder, or urinary bladder furnishes valuable information. The same is true if blood escapes from the bowel or bladder.

Foreign bodies, especially clothing, must be re-

* Brit. Jour. Surg., iv.

moved at whatever cost. If left behind, it is praetically a sentence of death.

Both Lockwood and his colleagues and Fraser and Drummond, in the same issue of the Journal, note that there may be a flaccid abdomen instead of rigidity. This is seen also in civil life, especially when shock and intestinal hemorrhage combine to exhaust the patient and before protective muscular rigidity has set in as a result of beginning peritonitis.

Wounds from *front to back*, as pointed out by Archibald,* are apt to have a favorable prognosis without operation, especially if on the right side, where the liver would be involved. If there be evidence of continuous hemorrhage, of course operation would be imperative.

Wounds from front to back, however, if in the midline, are apt to be very dangerous, as the great vessels [and the spine] may be involved.

Abdominal wounds from *side to side*, as a rule, are far more dangerous on account of the greater danger to the viscera. Wounds in the lower abdomen are more dangerous than those in the upper abdomen.

In his opinion peritonitis is not so frequent a cause of death as are shock and paralytic ileus causing obstruction. For the latter condition pituitrin is given.

* Canadian Med. Assoc. Jour., April, 1917.

It should be given *not* subcutaneously but intravenously or intramuscularly. Then he has found it very effective. If pituitrin fails, eserin may succeed in some cases.

The small intestine may exhibit multiple wounds, not only as in civil life, by multiple perforations from a single missile, but in this war especially from multiple missiles from exploded shell or shrapnel, to say nothing of additional wounds elsewhere in the body (*cf.* p. 67). One excellent piece of advice is given by Fraser and Drummond, and advocated also by others. First, determine how many wounds of the intestine there are, their extent and locality, before deciding on the proper treatment. Identify the cecum and then trace the small intestine from there upward. "As each perforation of the gut is exposed it is wrapped up in a small moist swab." The tape attached to the swab "is slipped through the mesentery and doubled twice around the gut." This prevents escape of the contents and additional infection, and gives one at a glance the means of judging what should be done. Special care should be taken not to overlook wounds of the posterior wall of the stomach and of the colon.

Since Crile has preached the "gospel of gentleness," no good surgeon will handle bowel or other viscera roughly or expose more than a foot or two at a time, nor dally with his operation. Speed, but never haste, is the rule. This is especially necessary when scores of cases may be urgently needing surgical relief.

As a rule, intestinal wounds susceptible to suture should be so treated even when there are several of them. Not seldom, however, a serious question will arise whether suture or resection should be resorted to. Most civil surgeons, I think, much prefer to avoid resection if possible. The authors of both the papers just referred to—in all, six authors, who between them had treated 800 abdominal wounds, an exceptional experience, which entitles their final judgment to special weight—and many others are decidedly of the same opinion. Fraser and Drummond go so far as to say that the only condition warranting resection is extensive damage to the mesentery or extravasation between the two layers of the mesentery at its attachment to the bowel where the latter is only partially covered by the peritoneum. Their reason is the profound shock which attends resection and which may easily turn the scale against the patient. Too many of us, in civil life, at least, do not give sufficient weight to this reason.

If resection has to be done, Lockwood and his colleagues prefer end-to-end suture; Fraser and

Drummond, and Bowlby prefer lateral anastomosis, so as to avoid distention of the proximal segment in end-to-end anastomosis. The latter do not seem to have tried what Lockwood and his associates recommend—before closing the abdomen, to milk the gut gently "from just above the distended area to just below the sutured area." Post-operative paralysis of the bowel—paralytic ileus—and distention, they assert, "practically never occurred" when this simple precaution was taken.

Lacerated kidneys may recover if not too widely injured. In these cases extensive experience and the resulting sound judgment are invaluable. Immediate nephrectomy is to be avoided, if possible, and to be resorted to (if then necessary) when the patient is in better condition. See an excellent paper on the kidney and ureter by Fullerton.* Before removing one kidney the actual presence of the other kidney should be always determined.

Irrigation and drainage of the peritoneal cavity are not commonly employed. Fraser and Drummond, however, particularly urge drainage in wounds of the colon, and especially posterior drainage, to avoid retrocolic infection. Obvious infection elsewhere may also require drainage.

* Brit. Jour. Surg., v, 248.

The Fowler position is desirable as soon as possible after the operation. If need be, drainage of the pelvis may be employed, but not probably for over twenty-four or thirty-six hours.

Sometimes morphin—which I have already commended as an initial measure for the relief of severe pain—is given in larger doses than is wise. This complicates recovery, especially by masking intra-abdominal symptoms.

According to Bowlby,* an operative recovery of 50 per cent. in present conditions is the best that one can expect—a great contrast to civil surgery! Hemorrhage and shock are the principal causes of this deplorable result. Hence again the need for quick transportation and prompt operation except in such deep shock as to forbid operation until reaction has been attained. If salines are to be used, it should be by *intravenous infusion*, for in deep shock little if any absorption takes place if it be given subcutaneously. But if serious hemorrhage then persists, operation to control it is the only possible hope. The pulse is of the greatest importance. Of 145 cases with a pulse over 120, only 16 recovered—a mortality of over 89 per cent. After thirty-six hours operation is rarely necessary.

* Brit. Med. Jour., June 2, 1917.

Bowlby gives the following table of results in 1038 cases treated during eighteen months:

Considered with view to operation....	1038
No operation advised..............	73
Total operations...................	965
Total operative mortality...........	53.9 per cent.
Total hollow viscera mortality.......	64.7 "
Stomach mortality*................	52.7 "
Small gut mortality*..............	65.8
Colon mortality*..................	58.7

* Uncomplicated by wound of any other hollow alimentary viscus.

BURNS

These are much more frequent in this war than in former wars because of the barbarous methods introduced by the Germans. Dr. Barthe de Sandfort greatly improved on the old paraffin dressings by a preparation which he named Ambrine, from the oil of amber mixed with the paraffin. I have seen a number of photographs of his cases and read papers published by those who have used it, and have no doubt as to the value of the treatment. Unfortunately, in absolute contravention of American medical ethics, he has kept the exact formula and the method of preparing it secret, and it can be obtained only from him or from the commercial company in Paris to whom he has divulged the secret.

Lieut.-Col. A. J. Hull, of the British Army,[*] after a series of experiments, has obtained a preparation which experience has shown to be superior to Ambrine. He calls it "No. 7 Paraffin." In the British Medical Journal, December 15, 1917, his latest formula is given:

[*] Brit. Med. Jour., January 13, 1917, p. 37.

Resublimed beta-naphthol... 0.25 per cent.
Eucalyptus oil.............. 2.00 "
Olive oil................... 5.00 "
Paraffinum molle (or vaselin). 25.00 "
Paraffinum durum.......... 67.75 "

The method of application is as follows: Wash the burn with a solution of acriflavin or proflavin 1 : 1000. This gives better results than saline solution. Dry it by fanning or by laying dry gauze on the surface. The paraffin mixture at 55° to 60° C. (131° to 140° F.) is then applied by a spray or by a broad camel's-hair brush, sterilized in wax and used very gently. It is important to apply a sufficiently thick layer of paraffin. At this temperature the layer is apt to be too thin.

"A thin layer of cotton-wool, cut the same size as the area of the burn, is placed over the wound after the first layer of paraffin has been applied. This layer of wool is covered with a second layer of paraffin. The wool is cut in thin sheets and pressed between layers of paper in order to obtain thin layers of wool. The dressing is completed by applying wool bandage. The burns are usually dressed daily (or later every second day). . . .

"Blisters are not interfered with in any way at the first dressing; the paraffin is applied after washing the burn. At the second dressing the dead layers of skin are cut away."

"Burns treated with No. 7 paraffin occasionally become sluggish. . . . We have, therefore, changed . . . to the scarlet-red paraffin when burns have become clean. . . . This treatment has resulted in great acceleration of healing" (Hull).

The formula for the scarlet-red paraffin is as follows:

Scarlet-red.................	0.2 per cent.
Eucalyptus oil..............	2.0 "
Olive oil...................	5.0 "
Adeps lanæ hydrosus........	4.0
Paraffinum molle...........	21.0
Paraffinum durum..........	67.8

This paraffin preparation has been employed to advantage also in "trench feet." Hurd[*] says that frozen fingers, toes, and ears "respond splendidly" to such treatment.

In the Journal of the American Medical Association for June 16, 1917, are two valuable articles by Sollmann and Beiter on the Paraffin Treatment of Burns which advance our knowledge considerably. Beiter especially has had a large experience in the treatment of burns in industrial works. Their conclusions are that the application of the ordinary melted paraffin to the wound is much too painful. They recommend, after cleansing, that the first application shall be the "Petrolatum Liquidum" (known com-

[*] Lancet, June 2, 1917, p. 855.

mercially as "Stanolind Liquid Paraffin"), which can be sprayed on the burn by the ordinary oil atomizer, or can be applied on a cotton swab. This is entirely painless. Then the cotton film is applied and the melted paraffin painted over it, etc., as usual.

Beiter says that "superficial burns heal more quickly by this treatment, but that when the tissues are destroyed in deep burns and scar tissue results, the scar tissue performs as scar tissue has performed since the beginning of time." Sir Anthony Bowlby, on the contrary, declares that the scars are "soft and supple and there is a marked absence of bad contractures." Others also have noted this advantage.

Risley,[*] in one of the best papers I have recently seen, has made a careful study of all cases of burn at the Massachusetts General Hospital for ten years, with a review of the recent literature. It well supplements the foregoing text.

In a severe burn the clinical picture is that of a profound toxemia affecting especially the kidneys, the gastro-intestinal tract, and the metabolism of the body. Pfeiffer, "Das Problem des Verbrühungstodes," holds that death comes from an auto-intoxication as a result of the destruction of proteid tissue at the site of the burn and the consequent absorption

[*] Boston Med. and Surg. Jour., September 13, 1917.

of the toxins. In experimental animals burned, removal of the burned tissue may be life saving. If the burned tissue is transplanted to another healthy animal, it may produce death with the same symptoms as if this animal had been burned. This is a very striking confirmation of the view that severe burns produce a profound toxemia.

As to treatment, the first question, says Risley, is not how to get clothes off and the dressings on, but *how much is the patient shocked and how can the shock be combated.* Sometimes, especially in the case of children, if the primary dressing is entirely carried out at once, the shock is increased to such a degree as to destroy life. The first thing to be given is a liberal dose of morphin, aided by subcutaneous salt infusion and rectal shock-enemata, and heat. If in half an hour the patient does not improve, then clothes and all he should be put into a continuous hot bath—90° to 110° F.,—of either saline or boric-acid solution. After the immersion the clothing may be cut away, not before. If he improves, say within a half-hour—then cut away the clothing gradually from the body, and place the patient naked exposed to the air in a room heated to 110° F. This plan has given by far the best results.

As to dressings, generally 15 per cent. picric acid

is applied in sections; or, if the burn is not extensive, and not beyond the second degree, the tincture of chlorid of iron is applied over the wound until the burned surface is well coated over and a dry protective layer formed. This is slightly painful for a short time. Patients beg for it later. The skin surface around the burned surface should be wiped off with alcohol to preserve asepsis. Paraffin mixtures he highly approves of. He regards the action of the paraffin as mechanical, and one of its special benefits is that the discharge floats the paraffin dressing off from the wound and so prevents its sticking to it.

No oily dressing whatever should be used. The dirty "Carron oil" dressing is sure to infect what, owing to the heat, is almost certainly at first a sterile wound, and should *never* be employed.

For moderate burns, especially in homes and in camps, the bicarbonate of soda, in the proportion of a teaspoonful to a pint of warm water, is one of the best.

Lee and Furness[*] commend the use of dichloramin-T. They employ only one layer of wide-meshed gauze, and spray the solution in the eucalyptus oil upon it. "No other dressing should be applied, and the usual technic of the open-air treatment of burns should be followed."

[*] Annals of Surg., January, 1918.

SHERMAN'S ATOMIZER FOR SPRAYING ANY MELTED PARAFFIN PREPARATION ON BURNS

Dr. W. O'Neil Sherman, Chief Surgeon of the Carnegie Steel Company, has devised an excellent apparatus for spraying any paraffin preparation on burns. It consists of an inner reservoir placed inside of an outer one. The space between the inner and the outer reservoir is filled with boiling water.

Directions for Use.—It is essential that the field to be treated be *entirely dry*, otherwise the patient will experience intense pain when the preparation comes in contact with the moist surface.

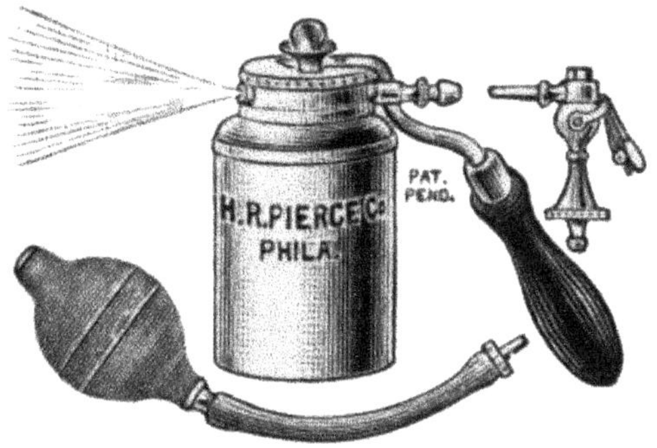

Fig. 53.—Sherman's atomizer for spraying any melted paraffin-base preparation for the treatment of burns and abrasions.

In order to dry it properly one or more layers of gauze should be lightly applied to the wet surface, followed, if possible, by a hot-air douche or by fanning.

Melt the preparation in a suitable pot, taking particular care that no liquid shall come in contact with it. Pour the melted preparation into the inner reservoir and close it tight. Pour boiling water into the water-jacket. Place the atomizer thus filled into an instrument sterilizer and keep it at the boiling temperature for about ten minutes. The preparation will then keep liquid for thirty minutes or more. The handle should be detached when placing the atomizer in the sterilizer. When finished, make sure to run a wire through the spray tube in order to free it from paraffin so that the instrument will be in proper condition for the next case.

The atomizer can be obtained from Harvey R. Pierce and Company, Philadelphia.

PERSONAL LETTERS

In the first edition of this book I published nine letters from surgeons of large experience. The defective mail service to and from France, and especially the exigencies of the war, have prevented the revision which I requested from the several authors of these early letters, excepting by Sir Anthony Bowlby, Major Joseph A. Blake, and Major George W. Crile. Not knowing how far the other writers might have changed their views, I did not feel authorized to reprint their earlier letters, for, as Cushing wrote me, "Times and opinions change and October 28, 1916, was in a previous existence."

I have been so fortunate as to secure new letters from Dr. Wm. S. Halsted as to the Carrel-Dakin treatment; a brief bibliography on the rehabilitation of crippled soldiers from Colonel R. Tait McKenzie, whose own remarkable work is so well known; and from Dr. Victor G. Heiser, relating his personal observations on the loading and unloading of hospital trains in Italy. In personal conversation Heiser was enthusiastic as to the entire medical and surgical methods of the Italians. He thinks them unsurpassed.

I have reprinted a few paragraphs from the earlier letter by Bowlby so that the marked changes in his views as a result of experience may be observed. These are especially marked in the increasing importance of early operation [and hence of the quickest possible transport]; in the treatment of shock; in the radical difference in the treatment of wounds of the chest; in the commendation of nitrous oxid and oxygen, and, above all, in the early and complete excision of all devitalized tissue with the greatest aseptic care, followed by immediate closure of the wound without drainage. This practically complete removal of the sources of infection is the latest triumph of Lister's principles.

Sir Anthony's tribute to our American surgeons is as agreeable as it is deserved.

LETTERS FROM SIR ANTHONY A. BOWLBY, BART.
(from the first edition, pp. 129–133)
British General Headquarters, France

. . . . .

"*The treatment of wounds* which today finds most favor is that known as Carrel's. This may be briefly summarized as excision of any *recently* wounded or dirty tissue and the subsequent irrigation of the wound by frequent instillation of 'Dakin's fluid.' In the British army the preparation known as 'Eusol' is often used instead of Dakin's fluid, from which it does not materially differ.

"Wounds already suppurating are *not* treated by *excision*.

. . . . .

"The *excision* of *damaged tissue* in all recently inflicted wounds is universally practised at the front whenever possible, *i. e.*, in all wounds of a serious or extensive nature.

"Fixation by efficient splints is always considered to be of very great importance.

"*Gas gangrene* may be caused by several different organisms, and is commonly due to a 'mixed infection.'

"In a great majority of all lacerated wounds gas will develop if they are left long enough undressed; especially if the wounded man lies out for a day or two. It is best prevented by the treatment described above.

"In many cases it is slight and local, and easily checked by free incision and subsequent drainage. The affected muscle-sheaths and fascia must be widely opened up, and if any one or two muscles are gangrenons, they must be excised.

"If a main artery is injured and the limb is affected by gas gangrene, amputation is necessary at once.

"In many compound fractures this same treatment is required.

"It is a noticeable fact that, however lacerated the face may be, gangrene never occurs in it or in the scalp, and hardly ever in the *neck*. I attribute this to the large blood-supply. I have never seen gas gangrene in any part of the *head*.

"*Gas* and gaseous crackling are often felt far above the area of *infection*, and it is a mistake to try and amputate above all *gas*.

. . . . .

"*Head Wounds at the Front.*—We avoid extensive operations and, with few exceptions, do not open an uninjured dura mater. It is very necessary not to move patients for about three weeks after operation, so that special accommodation is required.

"*Chest.*—Rest in bed and small doses of morphin for all and no tapping of effusion for several days.

"Subsequently, if there is a large hemothorax, either—(*a*) tap; (*b*) tap and replace with oxygen; or (*c*) if septic, excise rib and drain. Most cases can travel safely to the base after three or four days in bed, and operative treatment is generally done there."

"*Abdomen.*—Our general practice is *to operate* if the patient is got in before thirty-six hours, and very many are actually got in within three or four hours after the injury.

"Operations are *not* done if the wound is *high up* and there is good reason to believe there is no injury to any *hollow* viscus, as evidenced by the absence of all symptoms and by the site of the wound. (Of course, this statement might require revision in any *single* case, but it will give you an idea of our practice.)

"Our recovery rate for several thousand operations is about 45 per cent., mostly lives saved.

"*Place for Operations at the Front.*—At the *field ambulances* we only operate to—(a) Stop bleeding. (b) Amputate hopelessly smashed limbs. (c) Dress bad fractures, etc., under anesthetics. All other operations are done in the 'Casualty Clearing Stations,' of which there are over 50 spread behind our whole front and all accessible to road or rail. Patients can be kept in these in moderate numbers for a week or two, and can be got into them from the field ambulances in about half-hour to one hour.

"*Anesthetics.*—'Shipway's' apparatus for warm ether vapor is very good. It conserves ether, and there is a complete absence of all secretions of mucus and saliva."

Sir Anthony Bowlby's Second Letter

October 15, 1917.

Since I last wrote to you, after the Somme Fight, we have had the experience of another year of war, and I hope that we have been able to treat our wounded of this year all the better for our experience of 1916. I will tell you in a few words in what way our practice has changed.

In the first place, the increasing *importance of early operation* has been recognized by a great increase in the staffs of our Casualty Clearing Stations. We have added both nurses and orderlies, as well as surgeons, and have arranged for the transference of reinforcements from one part of the army to another of "surgical teams," each consisting of—a surgeon, an anesthetist, a nursing sister (who acts as assistant surgeon) and a trained theater orderly. You will be interested to learn that the "Battle of Flanders" or "The Third Battle of Ypres" afforded the first opportunity for appointing "Teams" from the United States units to serve on the staffs at the front in British Casualty Clearing Stations. They found there, not only surgeons from Great Britain itself, but also "teams" from Canada, Australia, New Zealand, and South Africa (a notable incident, I think!) and no more harmonious gathering could be imagined. But it was the advent of all this aid that enabled us *to save one man out of every three wounded brought to the operating theaters*, with the result that bad gas gangrene was hardly seen and that the comparative loss of lives and of limbs was very small. The results were altogether far in advance of anything we have known in our other battles.

We also made special efforts to treat "shock" on a more extensive scale than before, and now all motor ambulance cars are heated from the exhaust, and at all hospitals at the front we have specially heated beds (or wards) for these cases. Great benefit has been derived from intravenous injections of solutions of bicarbonate of soda (3 to 4 per cent.) and still more by transfusion of one or two pints of blood. We owe much of the latter practice to the previous experience of our American colleagues, and by the giving of blood many bad cases have passed from the "inoperable" state into the "operable," while other patients have been saved by a timely transfusion after operation has been done. We have also extended our use of nitrous oxid and oxygen as *the* anesthetic in cases of shock. There is no doubt at all but it is by far the best of them all.

The great improvement is in the treatment of our

chest wounds. Many we still leave without operation, except that we treat all wounds of the chest *wall* by just the same excision operations which we practise in all large wounds of the other parts of the body and limbs. But we also operate now on all cases where very large fragments are lodged and where bone fragments are driven into the lung, and we find that we can handle the lung with impunity, and that no special "atmospheric pressure" conditions are required. After operation all these wounds are completely closed by suture of the pleura and of the skin.

You ask me for my experience of the Carrel-Dakin, the Sir Almroth Wright, the dichloramin-T, and the Bipp methods.

Well, I have just the same opinions of the first two as when I last wrote to you. The Carrel-Dakin is *the best* method of all, and the hypertonic saline of Wright is nowhere in regular use at either the base or the front. It has been completely superseded by other and better methods.

Dichloramin-T I have only seen used in a few cases, and in oily solutions, for we could not obtain it until quite lately. The fresh wounds treated by it did not seem to do well, but for granulating wounds I think it is good, although irritating to the skin.

We want further experience before coming to any decision.

Bipp is in my opinion good, but it has been brought into some disrepute by zealous disciples who have used it in such excessive quantities that poisoning by bismuth or iodoform has occurred in a good many cases. It should be gently rubbed into the wounded surfaces, and then all that can be rubbed off with gauze should be removed before the wound is dressed.

It is, however, quite certain that the most important treatment is the early excision of all soiled and damaged tissue as far as possible, and where this can be done within twelve hours of injury, *a very large percentage of all the wounds can be closed by primary suture* if they are not very extensive or associated with bad fractures. At one C. C. S. we successfully closed 67 per cent. of all wounds, and at several other C. C. S. we have had similar success. I think, therefore, we shall soon suture the great majority of all recent wounds. In wounds older than twelve hours it is more difficult to obtain sufficiently aseptic conditions for primary suture, and it is especially in these that some sort of antiseptic treatment is of use. Opinions differ as to the best antiseptic agents, but I have no doubt at all that the Dakin solution and the Carrel method are the best means we at present possess for the sterilization of septic wounds, and I have no doubt at all that the antiseptic agent as such is of use as well as the method of using it.

Flavine in solution of 1 : 1000 has proved to be good in the treatment of recent wounds at the time of operation, but it is certainly not good for grannlating wounds.

Secondary suture is the objective of the surgeon if primary suture is not possible, and, as to the time to perform this, we are guided by the principles laid down by Carrel. Where large areas of skin have been destroyed, plastic operations and skin-grafting are of the greatest service. They are especially necessary in many shell wounds of the face.

LETTER FROM MAJOR JOSEPH A. BLAKE, M.R.C., U. S. ARMY

Paris, 12th January, 1918.

I am becoming more and more convinced that the principles of wound treatment in vogue in America before the war are substantiated by the experience here. In other words, the needlessness, even the harmfulness, of chemical sterilization (antisepsis) is becoming more evident, and particularly the danger of substituting chemical treatment for operative mechanical cleansing.

The best results I have observed and the best reported results have been in those services where an early (within twelve hours from the reception of the wound) operation is performed, and the lacerated tissues and foreign bodies removed (épluchage), leaving the wound surrounded by healthy living tissue. The wound is then immediately sutured; or if there is a reasonable doubt that the infecting agents have not been entirely eradicated, or if the patient has to be at once evacuated to another hospital, the wound is left open with a simple dry protective dressing until the third day, when, if there is no general or local evidence of infection, it is sutured. The interesting point is that if the wound is evidently infected and cannot be sutured, apparently more rapid and satisfactory disinfection of the wound is obtained by autosterilization; namely, by leaving the wound to itself, and not using any form of chemical substance other than a good scrubbing of the skin about the wound and the wound edges, with soap and water, and removing the soap with ether and afterward painting the skin and wound with iodin, to prevent the ingrowth of staphylococci. By this method 98 per cent. of wounds of the soft parts and about 80 per cent. of the fractures are successfully sutured and closed in two weeks. The fractures of the thigh, probably on account of the gross lesions of the muscles, are the most troublesome, and few surgeons have the temerity to close the wounds by immediate suture.

Perhaps the most interesting and greatest progress made has been in the surgery of wounds of the joints. Not only is the treatment by an early operation, as has just been described, almost uniformly successful, the joints being almost immediately closed; but when infection occurs and there is suppuration, the proper treatment seems to be simple evacuation of the pus, lavage of the joint, and either closure or leaving the joint open *without drains*. Just as I insisted fifteen years ago that the insertion of drains into a suppurating abdomen was useless, and even harmful if the sources of infection had been removed, so in the treatment of suppurating joints the same has been proved. We must admit now, from what we have seen, that the joints possess nearly, if not quite, the power of the peritoneum to sequestrate and eliminate infection.

Another interesting observation in regard to the surgery of the joints is that excellent results can be obtained by immediate mobilization and use of the joints. C. Wilhelms, of Brussels, is insistent that immediate mobilization affords the best results. He makes his patients who have wounds of the knee or ankle walk in three or four days. Whether he is right, I think, still remains to be seen.

I see no reason to change the views I expressed to you in my former letter as to the relative value of the Wright, Carrel-Dakin, and Bipp treatments, except that I believe that the treatment furnished by nature is better than them all, and we can aid and supplement nature better by removing the pabulum for the bacteria, and preventing the entrance of more, than by modifying the wound secretions by chemicals in solution or in mass.

What we must do is to put our best operating surgeons in our most advanced hospitals, and, in short, do all in our power to eliminate the causes of infection and the devitalized tissues upon which alone most bacteria can thrive.

LETTER FROM MAJOR GEORGE W. CRILE, M.R.C., U. S. ARMY

December 1, 1917.

. . . . I would like to say, first, that the practice of giving large doses of morphin to a seriously injured man who is to be transported is of very great importance. It protects him against further shock and the effects of the loss of food and drink; but if there is cyanosis, morphin should be withheld until the cyanosis has cleared.

I have not been able to form any conclusion as to the best method of treating gas gangrene, as all methods have proved so ineffectual. Of course, when it is to save the life of the patient, there is quick amputation, leaving the stump wide open, but this will lead to many needless amputations. The prevention of gas gangrene by early wound excision is well established.

Good results are being obtained by the Carrel-Dakin method; by Bipp; by eusol; and by dichloramin-T, but the primary consideration is early excision-revision,* physiologic rest, and good sound practical surgery.

Letter from Dr. William S. Halsted

Baltimore, December 14, 1917.

We were most fortunate in having with us last winter Dr. Joseph S. Lawrence, who for several months had been in charge of the bacterial work of the American Ambulance at Neuilly and had thoroughly familiarized himself with the details of the new antiseptic work. Dr. Lawrence made all of our bacterial counts and carefully supervised the techni-

* See footnote, p. 76.

cal details of the wound-treatment. We were able to confirm unqualifiedly the claims made for the method by Carrel and Dehelly, Depage, Tuffier, Debaisieux, Lagasse, and some others.

At the outset of our work with the Dakin-Daufresne solution we repeated on the human subject the experiments made by Carrel on dogs at the Rockefeller Institute.* Our patients readily consented to the experiments, which consisted merely in the removal of two squares of skin at symmetric points on the abdomen and observing the process and rate of healing under various contrasted conditions. The square defect on one side of the abdomen would be treated with the Dakin solution, and on the other either without an antiseptic or with naphthalin, blue ointment, nitrate of silver, *et al.* The healing under the Dakin solution was marvelously rapid, and the results so uniform that we accepted it as a standard for comparison with other methods, such as dry scab, moist blood-clot, dry cell, grafts deprived of epithelium and applied inside out, etc. Although not quite prepared to report our results, we can confidently affirm that the granulating wounds treated with the Dakin solution healed much more rapidly than any treated by other antiseptics.

* Jour. Amer. Med. Assoc., December 17, 1910.

Are you not surprised to note the absence of any reference to dead spaces in the writings either of those who extol or those who condemn the Carrel method? We know, of course, as Moynihan has emphasized in a recent paper, that fresh wounds of soft parts may, after scrupulous toilet, and without the employment of antiseptics, be closed with a fair prospect of healing by first intention; and we have frequently observed that even after amputation through infected tissues the undrained wound may heal *per primam*, provided that no dead space is left. If a dead space cannot be avoided without prejudicing the vitality of the tissues used to occlude it, the apposed soft parts may still unite primarily if the dead space at the end of the sawed-off bone is drained.

Having convinced myself of the remarkable effect of the Dakin-Daufresne solution upon infected wounds, I cherished the hope that possibly involucral cavities, if sterilized to the required degree, might, after closure, fill with granulations before the inhibited organisms would recover sufficiently to defeat the healing process. As every surgeon knows to his mortification, cases of osteomyelitis in which the sequestrum has or has not been removed may go from clinic to clinic for twenty years or more in the hope of having their fistulous tracts healed. It would, therefore, be a great boon to both patient and surgeon if by the Carrel method the old involucral cavities could be healed.

In four cases last year Dr. Dandy, our resident surgeon, irrigated for from twenty-five to thirty days with the Dakin solution, according to the Carrel method, the properly prepared involucral cavities, and then, the microörganisms having been reduced for six or more days to about 1 in 10 fields (the counts were made by Dr. Lawrence), the soft parts were trimmed and the wounds closed. For about six weeks in one case, eight weeks in two cases, and three weeks in a fourth the wounds remained closed and without evidence of revivement of the bacteria. Then the tissues became slightly inflamed and the wounds opened.

In a fifth case a fracture of the operatively reduced involucrum occurred and the fragments were wired together. In this instance the Carrel irrigation was continued for about two months—until the bony cavity had filled and the wound healed. Now, six months later, the wound is still firm and the fracture united.* So, too, in circumscribed bone abscesses, thanks to the care and interest of Dr. Dandy and

* Fancy what the result would have been in this case had the wound not been sterilized.

Dr. Lawrence, we have had admirable results with the method when the irrigation was continued until the cavity became filled with the new tissue.

Evidently, in the unsuccessful cases, the bony cavities with eburnated involucral walls produced granulations so slowly that the inhibited organisms recovered before the dead spaces became filled with living tissue. Thus the Carrel method will fail if the dead space is too large or its walls are too feeble to furnish sufficient granulation tissue in the required time. Dead spaces, and not alone devitalized bone or soft parts, must surely be a contributing cause of the failure of the Carrel method in many cases of compound fracture. Even in amputations the dead space between the end of the bone and the muscles might be responsible for the defeat of the surgeon's best efforts. Granulation tissue must fill the empty space before the bacteria in its fluid contents revive, otherwise the wound will break down. The walls of an infected dead space, enlarged from exudate or perhaps from hemorrhage, become tense and relatively devitalized, and thus the infection may spread to parts of the wound which have healed, and beyond. One should not demand the impossible from the Carrel-Dakin treatment.

In civil practice we should, I think, sterilize every

granulating wound, whether an abscess, sinus, or superficial ulcer; and attempt the sterilization of fistulæ. Surgeons will ultimately appreciate the magnitude of the lessons taught by Carrel, chief of which is that wounds may be practically sterilized by the constant contact of mild antiseptics. The contributions of Dakin are of almost equal importance, and indicate that it is chiefly the chemist to whom we must now look for further developments in the treatment of wounds in general.

Antiseptics in the Aseptic Period.—In the Surgical Clinic of the Johns Hopkins University we have never abandoned the use of chemical antiseptics. The surgeon who has lived in the days before Listerism needs no modern proof of their value. So far back as 1884 we had irrefutable confirmation of Carrel's view of the inhibitive action of mild antiseptic solutions. Gonorrhea was promptly cured by frequent irrigations of very large quantities (3000 c.c.) of solutions of the bichlorid of mercury as weak as 1 : 50,000, or even 1 : 100,000. The strength of the solution could be gradually increased to 1 : 20,000. From day to day we noticed the rapid diminution in the number of the Neisser cocci.

Since the first years of the Johns Hopkins Hospital the treatment of our infected joints has been as follows: An Esmarch bandage is applied above the affected joint to prevent absorption of the antiseptic; the joint is opened freely, flushed with the antiseptic solution for five or ten or even fifteen minutes, and then closed. If necessary, the procedure is repeated in a few days, and then perhaps again. The results in these cases alone should convince one of the value of antiseptics.

Further proof (if, indeed, fresh proof were needed) of their action we have from year to year in the results of the blood-clot treatment of old involucral cavities. These cavities are cleaned with meticulous care. Everywhere, both in bone and soft parts, only freshly cut surfaces remain as walls of the dead space. Pure carbolic acid is poured freely into the cavity (formalin may be as good or better) and scrubbed over all the raw surfaces for several minutes. Then for a prolonged period the wound is flushed with gallons of a corrosive sublimate solution—1 : 1000. The wound is loosely closed with a buried continuous wire suture, the Esmarch bandage removed, and the cavity allowed to fill with blood. Many layers of silver-foil are laid over the line of the suture, and over this the paper. The wound should not be investigated for two or three weeks unless there is reason to believe that the clot has broken down from infection.

LETTER FROM DR. VICTOR G. HEISER
Of the International Health Board of the Rockefeller Foundation

January 24, 1918.

Loading and Unloading Hospital Trains in Italy

"Transferring the wounded by hospital trains is accomplished in a very expeditious and systematic manner in Italy. Before the hour of departure all patients are given any required medical or surgical attention. Those who are able to walk are properly dressed, and their belongings, clinical records, etc., are assembled at the bedside. The more serious cases and those requiring special treatment are often grouped in separate cars. Sometimes such patients are given numbers, all holding like numbers being placed in the same car. At many hospitals the train backs directly into the hospital grounds, close to the wards, so that only a minimum amount of walking or stretcher service is required. At a given signal the loading begins in a systematic manner and is often completed and the train started within *thirty minutes*.

"The detraining is also done quickly and without confusion. At Rome, for instance, a freight station has been renovated and is used for this purpose. Upon the arrival of the train the patients are immediately carried into the station. A large force of Red Cross nurses and Sisters of Charity supply them with hot drinks and simple food. A force of nurses from the different hospitals to which the patients are to be sent are also at the station. The patients are rapidly assorted according to their particular injury or disease, and are sent to the hospital set aside for that purpose. Street-car tracks have been extended to the station, and all cases able to sit up are assisted to the waiting street-cars. The remainder of the patients are carried to the ambulances.

"The expeditiousness, the lack of confusion, and the absence of the appearance of haste are most striking."

BRIEF BIBLIOGRAPHY ON THE REHABILITATION OF CRIPPLED SOLDIERS KINDLY FURNISHED BY

MAJOR R. TAIT McKENZIE, R.A.M.C.

1. McKenzie: "Reclaiming the Maimed," Macmillan & Co., 1918.

The following papers are also by Major McKenzie:

2. "The Treatment of Convalescent Soldiers by Physical Means," Proceed. Royal Soc. of Med. (Surgical Section), 1916, pp. 31–62.

3. "The Making and Remaking of a Fighting Man," Physical Educ. Rev., March, 1917.
4. "The Treatment of Nerve, Muscle, and Joint Injuries by Physical Means," Canad. Med. Assoc. Jour., December, 1917.
5. Mennell: "Massage in the After Treatment of the Wounded," Lancet, October 2, 1915.
6. R. Fortesque Fox: "Physical Remedies for Disabled Soldiers."
7. A Bibliography of the War Cripple, compiled by Douglas C. McMurtrie, at the Red Cross Institute for Crippled and Disabled Men, 311 Fourth Avenue, New York City, will give many more titles.
8. American Journal of Care for Cripples. New York. Edited by Douglas C. McMurtrie.
9. A number of books and articles are cited in an editorial in the Journal of the American Medical Association for March 30, 1918, p. 927.

See also the Orthopedic Bibliography, page 60.

APPENDIX

The "Cotton-Process" Ether

While the proof-sheets were being corrected my attention was called to a paper by Dr. W. G. Hudson, Medical Director of the DuPont Powder Works in Wilmington, Del., published in the New York Medical Record of March 16, 1918. It was on "Cotton-Process Ether," *i. e.*, ether made by the process of Dr. James H. Cotton, of McGill University. Cotton's paper appeared in the Canadian Medical Association Journal of September, 1917.

Dr. Cotton believes that, as Hudson expresses it, "perfectly pure ether, for the manufacture of which an entirely new process had to be devised, is not an anesthetic at all, but produces, upon inhalation, merely a transitory stimulation similar to that from alcohol. Commercial anesthesia ether is by no means pure, but contains two sets of impurities, one of which produces the anesthesia, which we have been attributing to the ether itself, and the other the undesirable after-effects, which have been so great a drawback to the administration of ether. He then proceeded to charge his chemically pure ether with only the desirable impurities, going beyond the proportions in which they exist in ordinary anesthesia ether. When this was done, not only were the undesirable after-effects eliminated, but it was found possible to produce an entirely new type of anesthesia, during which the patient can be maintained in a condition in which all sensation is abolished, but in which he is perfectly conscious, can carry on a conversation intelligently, and can even walk about, although rather unsteadily. If the amount administered is reduced, sensation begins to return, while if it is pushed, the condition passes over into the ordinary surgical anesthesia, with loss of consciousness but without any intervening stage of excitement."

Cotton believes that the impurity which produces anesthesia is a gas similar to ethylene. The other is also a gas not yet synthetized, to which are probably due the nausea, headache, etc., following anesthesia by the ordinary commercial ether.

Dr. Hudson has been good enough to promise me a small quantity of this "new ether," which I shall ask the surgeons at the Jefferson Hospital to investigate. Of course it is quite too early as yet to express an opinion upon the unexpected and novel statements by Cotton and Hudson. Only after the chemists have had their "inning" and after the new ether has been tested by a number of surgeons, will it be possible and proper to formulate a well-considered judgment; certainly it is to be hoped that Cotton has made a real and valuable discovery.

Anesthesia During Dressing of Wounds

I find also in the "Military Surgeon" for April, 1918, on page 485, the following method of relieving soldiers from the severe pain which attends the dressing of certain wounds:

"In the dressing of painful wounds a very valuable method of anesthetizing the patient is used without danger, even though required daily. The formula of the anesthetic is as follows: Ethyl chlorid, 5 c.c.; chloroform, 1 c.c.; ether, 24 c.c. A piece of flannel cloth is saturated with the entire amount and placed over the patient's face; this is covered with another piece of flannel, and this in turn is covered with oiled silk containing a small aperture, fitting over the nostrils. This is tied around the patient's face with a bit of tape or rubber tubing. The anesthesia produced will last for ten minutes, and the dressing can be started on the second breath. This anesthesia is apparently devoid of danger, is not accompanied by unpleasant complications, is followed by no deleterious after-effects, and is welcomed by the patient."

INDEX

ABDOMINAL cavity, chest wounds involving, 208
wounds, 220
  Archibald on, 225
  Banksmith on, 220
  Bowlby on, 229
    letter on, 243
  Fowler, position in, 229
  Fraser and Drummond on, 225
  from back, 223
  from front to back, 225
  from side to side, 225
  Hughes on, 221
  importance of early treatment, 221
  intravenous saline infusion in, 229
  irrigation and drainage in, 228
  Jordan on, 220
  judging course of missile in, 222
  Lockwood on, 224
  morphin in, 229
  Rees on, 221
  Robinson on, 220
  shock from, 23
  Wallace on, 220, 221
  Walters on, 220
  Webb and Milligan on, 224
Abduction frame, Jones', for fracture of femur, 57
Acriflavine, 76
Adhesive plaster extension in fractures, 52
  Sinclair's glue for, 52, 56
    modification, 56

Adrenalin in shock, 26
Advanced dressing station, functions, 33
Aid post, regimental, functions of, 30
Alkaline drinks to prevent shock, 34
Aluminum splint for fractures of humerus, 52
Ambrine in burns, 231
Ambulance, automobile, method of heating, 42
  value of, 42
  railway trolley, 43, 44
    overhead, 44
  service, automobile, Thorn on, 37
Amputations, bipp treatment after, 121
  soap-and-water treatment, 72
  Tuffier on, 84
Anaphylaxis in tetanus, 148
Anesthesia during wound dressing, 264
  local, in head wounds, 191
Anesthetics, Bowlby's letter on, 243
Antisepsis in war wounds, 75
Antiseptics, Halsted's letter on, 257
  in prophylactic treatment of tetanus, 152
Antitoxin in tetanus, 147
  intramuscular injection, 157
  intrathecal injection, 158, 164
  intravenous injection, 157
  subcutaneous injection, 157
  prophylactic, in gas gangrene, 174
Archibald on abdominal wounds, 225
  on head wounds, 182

INDEX

Archibald and MacLean on shock, 36
Arm splint, Bowlby's, 49, 50
    Clarke's, 49, 50
    Thomas', in fractures of leg, 51
Armor, steel, return to use of, 18
Arthritis, prevention of, in joint wounds, 214
Asepsis in war wounds, 75
Ashhurst and John on tetanus, 145
Automobile ambulance, method of heating, 42
    value of, 42

BACILLUS aërogenes capsulatus, 166
    of Welch, 166
    perfringens, 166
    Reading, Donaldson and Joyce, 77
Balkan splint, 60
Banksmith on abdominal wounds, 220
Barges, hospital, 45
Barling on Carrel-Dakin treatment, 80
Bashford on excision of wounded tissue, 66
Bayliss on treatment of shock, 26
Beiter and Sollman on paraffin treatment in burns, 233
Bibliography on crippled soldiers, 260
    on fractures, 60
    orthopedic, 60
Bipp treatment, 118
    after amputations, 121
    after cerebral hernia, 121
    Bowlby's letter on, 247
    for suppurating sinuses, 120
    in gunshot fractures, 120
    ingredients used, 110
    objections to, 121
    preventing poisoning in, 119
    redressing in, 120

Bipp treatment, surgical principle of, 118
    technic, 119
Blake, Major Joseph A., letter from, 248
    on joint wounds, 250
    on wound sterilization, 249
Blankets, dry, method of carrying, 31
    method of wrapping patient in, 32
Bleaching powder and sodium carbonate method for Dakin's solution, 91
    titration of, for Dakin's solution, 923
Blood-pressure, critical level, 22
    in shock, 23
Borden on Carrel-Dakin method, 86
Bowlby, Sir Anthony A., letters from, 240, 244
    arm splint, 49, 50
    on abdominal wounds, 229, 243
    on anesthetics, 243
    on bipp treatment, 247
    on burns, 234
    on Carrel-Dakin treatment, 240, 246
    on chest wounds, 242, 246
    on dichloramin-T, 246
    on flavine, 248
    on gas gangrene, 168, 241
    on head wounds, 184, 242
    on infected wounds, 69
    on intestinal wounds, 221
    on joint wounds, 210
    on liver wounds, 222
    on shock, 35, 245
    on treatment of wounds at front, 41
Bowling on tetanus, 148
Brain, penetrating wounds of, indications for operation, 187, 188
British General Research Committee to Investigate Shock, 28

INDEX

Bruce on tetanus, 146
Bull and Pritchett's antitoxin in gas gangrene, 174
Bullet and shell wounds, proportion of, 62
Burns, 231
  ambrine in, 231
  Bowlby on, 234
  carron oil in, 236
  dichloramin-T in, 236
  Lee and Furness on, 236
  No. 7 paraffin in, 231
  paraffin in, Beiter and Sollmann on, 233
  Pfeiffer on, 234
  Risley on, 234
  Sherman's paraffin atomizer in, 237
  sodium bicarbonate in, 236
  tincture of chlorid of iron in, 236
  toxemia in, 235
  treatment, 235

CABOT on standardized stretchers, 43
Caldwell on stereofluoroscopy for localization of foreign bodies, 141
Cannon on shock, 29
Cannula and trocar method of localizing foreign bodies, 136
Carbolic acid in tetanus, 160
Carbon dioxid respiration for shock, 24
  apparatus for, 27
  technic, 27
Carrel on excision of wounded tissue, 66
  on soil infection of wounds, 68
Carrel and Du Noüy, planimeter of, 106–108

Carrel-Dakin method, 76, 86
  after-care, 102
  apparatus for, 95–98
  Barling on, 80
  Borden on, 86
  Bowlby's letters on, 240, 246
  chloramin paste in, 87
  disadvantages of, at overflow times, 19
  Gibson on, 81
  glass tubes for, 96
  Halsted's letter on, 253
  in empyema in chest wounds, 205
  in penetrating wounds, 100
  in superficial wounds, 100
  in suppurating wounds, 99
  in through-and-through wounds, 101
  instillation tubes in, introduction, 99
  Lee and Furness on, 83
  materials necessary, 95
  objections to, 109
  preparing wounds for, 97
  reunion of wound in, 104
  solutions, 87–93
  special training for, 86
  systematic bacteriologic examination in, 103
  technic of dressing, 95, 96
  Welch on, 79
Carron oil in burns, 236
Casualty clearing station, functions, 41
Cerebral hernia, bipp treatment after, 121
Chase on multiple shell wounds, 67
  on plaster-of-Paris casts, 58, 60
Chest, stove-in, 207
  Lockwood and Nixon on, 207
  wounds, 199
    Bowlby's letter on, 242

INDEX

Chest wounds, Depage on, 209
  dyspnea in, 200
  empyema in, treatment, 205
  hemorrhage in, 201
    treatment, 204
  hemothorax in, 201
    treatment, 205
  immobility in, 203
  infection in, 199
  involving abdominal cavity, 208
  mortality in, 208
  Moynihan on, 206
  open, 200
  operative treatment, 206
  penetrating, 199
    treatment, 203
  thoracentesis in, 202
  traumatopnea in, 200
    treatment, 203
  Tuffier on, 205
  usual missiles in, 199
  Wilkinson and Gask on, 200
  with lodged missiles, treatment, 204
Chloramin-T paste in Carrel-Dakin method, 87
  preparation of, 93
Chlorazene, 94
Chlorin and sodium carbonate method for Dakin's solution, 90
Clarke's arm splint, 49, 50
Cloth fragments in shell wounds, 63
Corrective orthopedics, 47
Cotton-process ether, Hudson on, 262
Craniocerebral wounds, 180
Crile, Major George W., letter from, 251
  on maggots in wounds, 73
  on mud wounds, 65
  on use of morphin, 60, 251
Crippled soldiers, bibliography on rehabilitation of, 260

Critical level of blood-pressure, 22
  in shock, 23
Cushing on head wounds, 179, 189

DAKIN's method of preparing dichloramin-T, 111
  solution, 87
    definition, 87
    McCartney and Mewburn on, 88
    preparation of, from chlorin and sodium carbonate, 90
    preparation of, methods, 89
    stronger solution, 92
    tests for alkalinity, 89
    titration of bleaching powder for, 93
Dakin-Carrel method. See *Carrel-Dakin method*
Daufresne chloramin-T paste, preparation, 93
Decompression in head wounds, 183
Delayed tetanus, 148, 153
Depage humerus splint, 51
  on chest wounds, 209
Dichloramin-T, 76, 111
  action of, 113
  Bowlby's letter on, 246
  clinical results of, 116
  Dakin's method of preparing, 111
  in burns, 236
  in old infected wounds, 115
  Lee and Furness on, 114
  oil spray for application of, 112
  stock solutions, 113
  technic of application, 114
Donaldson and Joyce on Reading bacillus, 77
Doubtful cases, observation wards for, 20
Drainage in abdominal wounds, 228

INDEX

Dressing station, advanced, functions, 33
  functions, 41
  wounds, anesthesia during, 264
Drummond and Fraser on abdominal wounds, 225
Du Noüy and Carrel, planimeter of, 106–108
Dyspnea in chest wounds, 200

Elbow, excision of, 217
Embolism, fat, shock caused by, 23
Empyema in chest wounds, treatment, 205
Epinephrin, action of, Meltzer on, 27
Épluchage, 249
Ether, Cotton-process, Hudson on, 262
Eupad, 85
Eusol, 85
Excisions of joints, primary, unwisdom of, 56
Exhaustion, effect of, on wound healing, 74
Extension in fracture by adhesive, 52

Fat embolism as cause of shock, 23
Femur, fracture of. See *Fractures of femur*
  shell-fractures of, shock from, 23
First-aid in front-line trenches, 29
  station, functions, 41
  waterproof sheet-blanket packet system for, 30
Flavine, 75
  Bowlby's letter on, 248
Fleming on gas infection, 166
Fluoroscope for localization of foreign bodies, 137

Foreign bodies, localization of, by x-rays, 123
  cannula and trocar method, 136
  Hirtz's compass for, 134
  parallax method, 130
  profondometer for, 130
  Strohl's method, 123
  fluoroscopy for, 137
  stereo-fluoroscopy for, 140
  removal of, 144
Fowler position in abdominal wounds, 229
Fractures, 46
  bibliography on, 59
  bipp treatment, 120
  extension in, by adhesive, 52
  of femur, 47
    abduction frame for, 57
    Jones on, 49
    special hospitals for, 47
  of humerus, aluminum splint for, 52
    Thomas splint for, 49, 50
  of leg, Thomas arm splint in, 51
  shell, of femur, shock from, 23
Fraser and Drummond on abdominal wounds, 225
Front-line trenches, first aid in, 29
Frostbite, paraffin in, Hurd on, 233
Furness and Lee on Carrel-Dakin treatment, 83
  on dichloramin-T, 114

Gamlen and Smith on head wounds, 182
Gangrene, gas, 166. See also *Gas gangrene*
  hospital, 177. See also *Hospital gangrene*
Gas gangrene, 166

INDEX

Gas gangrene, bacterial cause, 166
  Bowlby on, 168
    letter on, 241
  guillotine amputation in, 173
  prophylactic antitoxin in, 174
  Taylor on, 171
  Tissier on, 167
  treatment, 171
  infection, 166
  Fleming on, 166
Gask and Wilkinson on chest wounds, 200
Gibson on Carrel-Dakin treatment, 81
  on tetanus, 146
Glue, Sinclair's, for adhesive plaster, 52
  modification, 56
Gooch's splint, 54
Goodwin on dressing wounds, 74
  diagram of zones of collection, evacuation and distribution of wounded in British Army, 40
Gray on head injuries, 194
  on joint wounds, 214
  salt pack treatment, 77
Guillotine amputation in gas gangrene, 173

HALSTED, Dr. William S., letter from, 252
  on antiseptics, 257
  on Carrel-Dakin treatment, 253
Haycroft's soap-and-water and primary suture treatment, 70
Head wounds, 179
  Archibald on, 182
  Bowlby on, 184
    letter on, 242
  cleaning track of missile in, 193
  Cushing on, 179, 189
  decompression in, 183

Head wounds, Gray on, 194
  gutter type, 182
  local anesthesia in, 191
  neurologic examination in, 190
  opening skull in, 193
  operating team to handle, 190
  Sargent on, 185, 187
  shaving scalp in, 191
  Smith and Gamlen on, 182
  syringe-catheter method of cleansing, 195
  three-legged incision in, 191
Heat, application of, to prevent shock, 29–34
Heel clip, Tapson's, 55
Heiser, Dr. Victor G., letter from, 259
  on transportation of wounded, 259
Hemorrhage in chest wounds, 201
  treatment, 204
Hemothorax in chest wounds, 201
  treatment, 205
Hernia, cerebral, bipp treatment after, 121
Hirtz's compass for localization of foreign bodies, 134
Holmes on shock, 36
Holmes and Sargent on decompression in head wounds, 183
Hospital barges, 45
  gangrene, 177
    Makins on, 177
    treatment, 178
  ships, 45
  trains, 45
Hospitals, special, for fractures of femur, 47
Hudson on Cotton process ether, 262
Hughes on abdominal wounds, 221
Hull's No. 7 paraffin for burns, 231
Humerus, fractures of, aluminum splint for, 52

INDEX

Humerus, fractures, Thomas splint for, 49, 50
  splint, Depage, 51
    Jones extension, 53
Hurd on paraffin in frost-bite, 233
Hypertonic salt solution treatment, Wright's, 77
Hypochlorite solution. See *Dakin's solution*

IMMOBILIZATION in chest wounds, 203
  in joint wounds, 213
  in wounds, Moynihan on, 45
Infection, gas, 166
  Fleming on, 166
Instillation tubes in Carrel-Dakin method, introduction of, 99
Intestinal wounds, Bowlby on, 221
    multiple, 226
    resection in, 227
Intra-abdominal wounds, dichloramin-T in, 116
Intramuscular injection of tetanus antitoxin, 157
Intrathecal injection of tetanus antitoxin, 158
    method of, 164
Intravenous injection of olive oil in shock, 23
  of tetanus antitoxin, 157
  saline infusion in abdominal wounds, 229
Iron, tincture of chlorid, in burns, 236
Irrigation in abdominal wounds, 228

JOHN and Ashhurst on tetanus, 145
Joint wounds, 210
    Blake's letter on, 250
    Bowlby on, 210

Joint wounds, Gray on, 214
  immobilization in, 213
  Jones on, 56
  prevention of arthritis in, 214
  resection in, 216
  with lodged missiles, 213
Joints, excision of, primary, unwisdom of, 56
Jones' abduction frame for fractures of femur, 57
  extension humerus splint, 53
  fracture splint, 54
  on fractures of femur, 49
  on joint wounds, 56, 216
  on orthopedics in war, 46
Jordan on abdominal wounds, 220
Joyce and Donaldson on Reading bacillus, 77

KIDNEYS, lacerations of, 228
Knee-joint, wounds of, amputation in, 219
  primary closure, 211
  soap-and-water and primary suture in, 72
  treatment, 218
Knee splint, Thomas', 53

LACERATIONS of kidneys, 228
Lee on shell wounds, 62
Lee and Furness on burns, 236
  on Carrel-Dakin treatment, 83
  on dichloramin-T, 114
Leg, fractures of, Thomas arm splint in, 51
Letter from Major Joseph A. Blake, 248
  from Major George W. Crile, 251
  from Dr. William S. Halsted, 252

272 INDEX

Letter from Dr. Victor G. Heiser, 259
Letters from Sir Anthony A. Bowlby, 240, 244
Liver wounds, Bowlby on, 222
Local anesthesia in head wounds, 191
Localization of foreign bodies by x-rays, 123
    cannula and trocar method, 136
    Hirtz's compass for, 134
    parallax method, 130
    profondometer for, 130
    Strohl's method, 123
    fluoroscopy for, 137
    stereo-fluoroscopy for, 140
Localized tetanus, 153
Lockwood on abdominal wounds, 224
Lockwood and Nixon on stove-in chest, 207

MacLean and Archibald on shock, 36
Maggots in wounds, 73
Magnesium sulphate in tetanus, 160
Makins on hospital gangrene, 177
McCartney and Mewburn on Dakin's solution, 88
Meltzer on action of epinephrin, 27
Mercurophen, 76
Mewburn and McCartney on Dakin's solution, 88
Milligan and Webb on abdominal wounds, 224
    on precedence in care of wounded, 21
    on removal of foreign bodies, 144
Montenovesi cranial forceps, 193
Morison's bipp treatment, 77, 118. See also *Bipp treatment*
Morphin in abdominal wounds, 229
    in first-aid treatment, 29

Morphin, use of, Crile on, 66, 251
Moynihan on chest wounds, 206
    on immobilization in wounds, 45
    on tetanus, 147
Mud wounds, Crile on, 65
Multiple shell and shrapnel wounds, 67
Muscles, hardening of, in tetanus, 156

New weapons of war, 62
Nixon and Lockwood on stove-in chest, 207

Observation wards for doubtful cases, 20
Oil spray for application of dichloramin-T, 112
Olive oil, intravenous injection, in shock, 23
Operating team to handle head wounds, 190
Orthopedics, corrective, 47
    in war, Jones on, 46
    preventive, 46
Osgood on splints in fractures, 50

Page's diagram of zones of collection, evacuation, and distribution of wounded in U. S. Army, 39
Page on transportation of wounded, 38
Paraffin in burns, Beiter and Sollmann on, 233
    in frost-bite, Hurd on, 233
    No. 7, in burns, 231
Parallax method of localizing foreign bodies, 130
Patient, method of wrapping in blankets, 32

INDEX

Penetrating wounds, Carrel-Dakin method in, 100
   of chest, 199
     treatment, 203
Pfeiffer on burns, 234
Pharyngeal muscle spasm in tetanus, 154
Planimeter of Carrel and du Noüy, 106-108
Plaster, adhesive, Sinclair's glue for, 52
Plaster-of-Paris casts, Chase on, 58, 60
Porter on shock, 22, 35
Preventive orthopedics, 46
Pritchett and Bull's antitoxin in gas gangrene, 174
Proflavine, 76
Profondometer for localizing foreign bodies, 133

Railway ambulance, trolley, 43, 44
   overhead, 44
Reading bacillus, Donaldson and Joyce on, 77
Rees on abdominal wounds, 221
Regimental aid post, functions of, 30
Removal of foreign bodies, 144
Resection in joint wounds, 216
Respiration, carbon dioxid, for shock, 24
     apparatus for, 27
     technic, 27
Risley on burns, 234
Robinson on abdominal wounds, 220

Salt pack treatment, Gray's, 77
Sandfort's ambrine treatment for burns, 231

Sargent on head wounds, 185, 187
Sargent and Holmes on decompression in head wounds, 183
Scalp, shaving of, in head wounds, 191
   wounds, 181
Shell and bullet wounds, proportion of, 62
   wounds, cloth fragments in, 63
   infection from, 62
   Lee on, 62
   multiple, 67
Shell-fractures of femur, shock from, 23
Sherman's paraffin atomizer in burns, 237
Ships, hospital, 45
Shock, 22
   adrenalin in, 26
   Bayliss on treatment, 26
   Bowlby on, 35
     letter on, 245
   British General Research Committee to Investigate, 28
   Cannon on, 29
   carbon dioxid respiration for, 24
     apparatus for, 27
     technic, 27
   critical level of blood-pressure in, 23
   fat embolism as cause of, 23
   from abdominal wounds, 23
   from multiple wounds through subcutaneous fat, 23
   from shell-fractures of femur, 23
   general treatment, 24
   Holmes on, 36
   intravenous injection of olive oil in, 23
   MacLean and Archibald on, 36
   Porter on, 22, 35
   prevention of, 30
     alkaline drinks for, 34

274 INDEX

Shock, prevention, application of heat for, 29-34
    intravenous injection of sodium bicarbonate for, 34
    room for treatment of, 24
Shoulder, excision of, 217
Sinclair's glue for adhesive plaster, 52
    modification, 56
Sinus, longitudinal, wounds of, 180
Sinuses, suppurating, bipp treatment, 120
Skull, opening of, in head wounds, 193
Smith and Gamlen on head wounds, 182
Soap-and-water and primary suture treatment of amputations, 72
    of wounds, 70
    of knee-joint, 72
Sodium bicarbonate in burns, 236
    intravenous injection, to prevent shock, 34
    carbonate and bleaching powder method for Dakin's solution, 91
    and chlorin method for Dakin's solution, 90
Soil infection of wounds, Carrel on, 68
Soldiers, crippled, bibliography on rehabilitation of, 260
Sollmann and Beiter on paraffin treatment in burns, 233
Splint, aluminum, for fractures of humerus, 52
    Balkan, 60
    Bowlby's arm, 49, 50
    Clarke's arm, 49, 50
    Depage humerus, 51
    Gooch's, 54
    Jones' extension humerus, 53
        fracture, 54
    Thomas' arm, in fractures of leg, 51

Splint, Thomas', for fractures of humerus, 49, 50
    knee, 53
Splints, standardized, 52
Steel armor, return to use of, 18
Stereofluoroscopy for localization of foreign bodies, 140
    Caldwell on, 141
Sterilization of wounds, Blake's letter on, 249
Stove-in chest, 207
    Lockwood and Nixon on, 207
Stretchers, standardized, Cabot on, 43
Subcutaneous fat, multiple wounds through, shock from, 23
    injection of tetanus antitoxin, 157
Superficial wounds, Carrel-Dakin method in, 100
Suppurating sinuses, bipp treatment, 120
    wounds, Carrel-Dakin method in, 99
Syringe-catheter method of cleansing head wounds, 195

Tapson's heel clip, 55
Taylor's (Kenneth) method of obtaining Bacillus of Welch in pure culture, 167
Taylor on gas gangrene, 171
Tetanus, 145
    anaphylaxis in, 148
    antitoxin in, 147
        intramuscular injection, 157
        intrathecal injection, 158
            method of, 164
        intravenous injection, 157
        subcutaneous injection, 157
    Ashhurst and John on, 145
    Bowling on, 148

INDEX

Tetanus, Bruce on, 146
  carbolic acid in, 160
  chronic forms, 158
  curative treatment, 165
    dosage, 159
  delayed, 148, 153
  diagnosis, 152
  Gibson on, 146
  hardening of muscles in, 154
  in trench feet cases, 151, 164
  incubation period, 146
  instruction to medical officers regarding, 163
  localized, 146, 153
  magnesium sulphate in, 160
  Moynihan on, 147
  precautions against, in operating, 151
  prophylactic treatment, antiseptics in, 152
    dosage in, 151
  protective inoculation against, 146
  reporting and care of cases, 161
  spasm of pharyngeal muscles in, 154
  specific treatment, 156
  surgical treatment of wound after appearance of, 161
  symptomatic treatment, 160
Thomas' arm splint in fractures of leg, 51
  knee splint, 53
  splint for fractures of humerus, 49, 50
Thoracentesis in chest wounds, 202
Thorn on Automobile Ambulance Service, 37
Three-legged incision in head wounds, 191
Through-and-through wounds, Carrel-Dakin method in, 101
Tissier on gas gangrene, 167

Toxemia in burns, 235
Trains, hospital, 45
Transportation of wounded, 37
  Heiser's letter on, 259
  Page on, 38
Traumatopnea in chest wounds, 200
Trench feet, tetanus in cases of, 151, 164
Trenches, front-line, first-aid in, 29
Tripod incision in head wounds, 191
Trolley railway ambulance, 43, 44
  overhead, 44
Tuffier on amputations, 84
  on chest wounds, 205

WALLACE on abdominal wounds, 220, 221
Walters on abdominal wounds, 220
  on observation wards for doubtful cases, 20
War, new weapons, 62
  orthopedic surgery in, Jones on, 46
  present, contrasted with preceding wars, 18
  huge numbers in armies, 19
Wards, observation, for doubtful cases, 20
Waterproof sheet-blanket packet system, 30
Webb and Milligan on abdominal wounds, 224
  on precedence in care of wounded, 21
  on removal of foreign bodies, 144
Welch bacillus, 166
  on Carrel-Dakin treatment, 79
Wilkinson and Gask on chest wounds, 200
Wounded, precedence in care of, 20
  Webb and Milligan on, 21

INDEX

Wounded, transportation of, 37
    Heiser's letter on, 259
    Page on, 38
Wounds, abdominal, shock from, 23
  antisepsis in, 75
  asepsis in, 75
  craniocerebral, 180
  devitalizing of surrounding tissues in, 65
  dressing of, anesthesia during, 264
    Goodwin on, 74
  effect of exhaustion on healing, 74
  excision of surrounding tissue in, Bashford on, 66
    Carrel on, 66
  immobility in, Moynihan on, 45
  infected, Bowlby on, 69
    Wright on, 69
  intra-abdominal, dichloramin-T in, 116
  joint, Jones on, 216
  maggots in, 73
  mud, Crile on, 65
  multiple, through subcutaneous fat, shock from, 23
  of abdomen, 220. See *Abdominal wounds*
  of brain, penetrating, indications for operation in, 187, 188
  of chest, 199. See also *Chest wounds*
  of head, 179. See also *Head wounds*
  of intestines, Bowlby on, 221
    multiple, 226
    resection in, 227
  of joints, 210. See also *Joint wounds*
  of knee-joint, amputation in, 219
    primary closure, 211
    soap-and-water and primary suture treatment, 72
    treatment, 218

Wounds of liver, Bowlby on, 222
  of longitudinal sinus, 180
  old infected, dichloramin-T in, 116
  penetrating, Carrel-Dakin method in, 100
  preparation of, for Carrel-Dakin method, 97
  ruthless excision in, 70
  scalp, 181
  shell and bullet, proportion of, 62
    cloth fragments in, 63
    infection from, 62
    Lee on, 62
    multiple, 67
  shrapnel, multiple, 67
  soap-and-water and primary suture treatment, 70
  soil infection of, 68
    Carrel on, 68
  sterilization of, Blake's letter on, 249
  superficial, Carrel-Dakin method in, 100
  suppurating, Carrel-Dakin method in, 99
  through-and-through, Carrel-Dakin method in, 101
  treatment at front, Bowlby on, 41
Wright hypertonic salt solution treatment, 77
  on wound infection, 69

X-RAYS, localization of foreign bodies by, 123
    cannula and trocar method, 136
    Hirtz's compass for, 134
    parallax method, 130
    profondometer for, 133
    Strohl's method, 127

Our books are revised frequently, so that the editions you find here may not be the latest. Write us about any books in which you are interested

GYNECOLOGY

and

OBSTETRICS

W. B. SAUNDERS COMPANY

West Washington Square   Philadelphia

9. Henrietta Street   Covent Garden, London

Our Handsome Complete Catalogue will be Sent on Request

Graves' Gynecology

Text-Book of Gynecology. By WILLIAM P. GRAVES, M. D., Professor of Gynecology at Harvard Medical School. Large octavo of 770 pages, with 425 original illustrations, many in colors. Cloth, $7.00 net.

TWO PRINTINGS IN FIVE MONTHS

This new work presents gynecology along new lines. An entire section is devoted exclusively to the *physiology* of the pelvic organs and to *correlated gynecology*—the relationship of gynecology to organs of *internal secretion*, breast, skin, organs of sense, digestion and respiration, blood, circulatory apparatus, abdominal organs, nervous system, bones, and joints. A special section is devoted to *enteroptosis*, intestinal bands, and movable kidney.

The second portion of the book is devoted to special gynecologic disease and is arranged particularly for the convenience of medical students. The first two parts (covering 500 pages) are entirely *non-surgical*, giving only drug and mechanical therapy and material invaluable to the general practitioner. The third part is exclusively a treatise on *surgical gynecology*, and includes profusely illustrated descriptions of those gynecologic operations that to the author seem most feasible. A number of new operations are given.   **Published May, 1916**

DeLee's New Obstetrics

Text-Book of Obstetrics. By JOSEPH B. DELEE, M. D., Professor of Obstetrics at Northwestern University Medical School, Chicago. Large octavo of 1087 pages, with 938 illustrations, 175 in colors. Cloth, $8.00 net.

Published August, 1915

SECOND EDITION

You will pronounce this new book the most elaborate, the most superbly illustrated work on Obstetrics you have ever seen. Especially will you value the 938 illustrations, all, with but few exceptions, original, and the best work of leading medical artists. Some 175 of these illustrations are in color. Such a magnificent collection of obstetric pictures—and with *really practical value*—has never before appeared in one book.

You will find the text extremely practical throughout. *Diagnosis* is featured, and the relations of obstetric conditions and accidents to general medicine, surgery, and the specialties are brought into prominence.

Regarding *Treatment:* You get here the very latest advances in this field, and you can rest assured every method of treatment, every step in operative technic, is just right. Dr. DeLee's twenty-one years' experience as a teacher and obstetrician guarantees this.

Worthy of your particular attention are the descriptive legends under the illustrations. These are unusually full, and by studying the pictures serially with their detailed legends you are better able to follow the operations than by referring to the pictures from a distant text—the usual method.

Prof. W. Stoeckel, *Kiel, Germany*

" Dr DeLee's Obstetrics deserves the greatest recognition. The whole work is of such sterling character through and through that it must be ranked with the best works of our literature."

Norris' Gonorrhea in Women

GONORRHEA IN WOMEN. By CHARLES C. NORRIS, M. D., Instructor in Gynecology, University of Pennsylvania. With an Introduction by JOHN G. CLARK, M. D., Professor of Gynecology, University of ·lvania. Large octavo of 520 pages, illustrated. Cloth, $6.50

Published May, 1913

Davis' Manual of Obstetrics

Manual of Obstetrics. By EDWARD P. DAVIS, M. D., Professor of Obstetrics in Jefferson Medical College. 12mo of 463 pages, with 171 original illustrations. Cloth, $2.25 net.

Published September, 1914

ORIGINAL ILLUSTRATIONS

Dr. Davis' manual is a concise text-book of exceptional value. Dr. Davis, himself a teacher of many years' experience, knows the requirements of such a work and has here supplied them. You get anatomy of the normal and abnormal bony pelvis, physiology of impregnation, anatomy of the birth canal in pregnancy, growth and development of the embryo. You get a full and clear discussion of pregnancy—its diagnosis, physiology, hygiene, pathology. You get the causes and treatment of labor, the physiology, conduct, pathology; the puerperal period—care of the mother and child; obstetric surgery, fetal pathology, mixed feeding, and medicolegal aspects of obstetric practice.

Davis' Operative Obstetrics

Operative Obstetrics. By EDWARD P. DAVIS, M. D., Professor of Obstetrics at Jefferson Medical College, Philadelphia. Octavo of 483 pages, with 264 illustrations. Cloth, $5.50 net.

Published September, 1911

INCLUDING SURGERY OF NEWBORN

Dr. Davis' new work on Operative Obstetrics is a most practical one, and no expense has been spared to make it the handsomest work on the subject as well. Every step in every operation is described minutely, and the technic shown by beautiful new illustrations. The section given over to surgery of the newborn you will find unusually valuable. It gives you much information you want to know—facts you can use in your work every day. There is an excellent chapter on anesthesia in obstetrics.

The Lancet, *London*

"The best and most interesting part of the book is the *summary of results* given at the end of the chapters and compiled from the author's own experience and from the literature."

Ashton's Practice of Gynecology

SIXTH EDITION—published October, 1916

The Practice of Gynecology. By W. EASTERLY ASHTON, M.D., LL.D., Professor of Gynecology at the Medico-Chirurgical College, Graduate School of Medicine, University of Pennsylvania. Octavo of 1097 pages, containing 1052 original line-drawings. Cloth, $6.50 net.

Among the important new matter may be mentioned the De Keating-Hart fulguration treatment, Coley's mixed toxins for sarcoma of the genito-urinary organs, the cutireaction of von Pirquet in the diagnosis of tuberculosis, "606" for syphilis, the hormone theory, the Fowler-Murphy treatment of suppurative peritonitis, tincture of iodin in sterilization, and Baldy's new round ligament operation for retrodisplacement. Nothing is left to be taken for granted, the author not only telling his readers in every instance what should be done, but also precisely *how to do it*. A distinctly original feature of the book is the illustrations, numbering 1058 line drawings made especially under the author's personal supervision.

From its first appearance Dr. Ashton's book set a standard in *practical* medical books; that he *has* produced a work of unusual value to the medical practitioner is shown by the demand for new editions.

Howard A. Kelly, M. D.,
Professor of Gynecologic Surgery, Johns Hopkins University

"It is different from anything that has as yet appeared. The illustrations are particularly clear and satisfactory One specially good feature is the pains with which you describe so many *details* so often left to the imagination"

Charles B. Penrose, M. D.,
Formerly Professor of Gynecology, University of Pennsylvania.

"I know of no book that goes so thoroughly and satisfactorily into all the *details* of everything connected with the subject. In this respect your book differs from the others."

George M. Edebohls, M.D.
Professor of Diseases of Women, New York Post-Graduate Medical School.

"I have looked it through and must congratulate you upon having produced a text-book most admirably adapted to *teach* gynecology to those who must get their knowledge, even to the minutest and most elementary details, from books."

Bandler's Medical Gynecology

Medical Gynecology. By S. WYLLIS BANDLER, M. D., Adjunct Professor of Diseases of Women, New York Post-Graduate Medical School and Hospital. Octavo of 790 pages, with 150 original illustrations. Cloth, $5.00 net.

Published February, 1914

THIRD EDITION—60 PAGES ON INTERNAL SECRETIONS

This new work by Dr. Bandler is just the book that the physician engaged in general practice has long needed. It is truly *the practitioner's gynecology*—planned for him, written for him, and illustrated for him. There are many gynecologic conditions that do not call for operative treatment; yet, because of lack of that special knowledge required for their diagnosis and treatment, the general practitioner has been unable to treat them intelligently. This work gives just the information the practitioner needs.

American Journal of Obstetrics
"He has shown good judgment in the selection of his data. He has placed most emphasis on diagnostic and therapeutic aspects. He has presented his facts in a manner to be readily grasped by the general practitioner."

Bandler's Vaginal Celiotomy

Vaginal Celiotomy. By S. WYLLIS BANDLER, M. D. Octavo of 450 pages, with 148 illustrations. Cloth, $5.00 net.

SUPERB ILLUSTRATIONS

The vaginal route, because of its simplicity, ease of execution, absence of shock, more certain results, and the opportunity for conservative measures, constitutes a field which should appeal to all surgeons, gynecologists, and obstetricians. Posterior vaginal celiotomy is of great importance in the removal of small tubal and ovarian tumors and cysts, and is an important step in the performance of vaginal myomectomy, hysterectomy, and hysteromyomectomy. Anterior vaginal celiotomy with thorough separation of the bladder is the only certain method of correcting cystocele.   January, 1911

The Lancet, London
"Dr. Bandler has done good service in writing this book, which description of all the operations which may be undertaken throughout a strong case for these operations."

Hirst's Obtetrics

New (8th) Edition

A Text-Book of Obstetrics. By BARTON COOKE HIRST, M. D., Professor of Obstetrics in the University of Pennsylania. Handsome octavo of 875 pages, with 716 illustrations. Ready in January, 1918.

The revision of the work for this edition was so thorough and complete that the book had to be entirely reset. Nothing has been omitted that could make this work a practical, valuable text-book embracing all the modern advances in the field. Among the new subjects included are the use of Dakin's solution and of the sunlight and open-air treatment of puerperal infections, a new chapter on various anesthesias in obstetrics, and another on the repair of injuries of the genital tract due to childbirth. The illustrations form one of the features of the book. They are numerous and most of them are original.

British Medical Journal

"The illustrations in Dr. Hirst's volume are far more numerous and far better executed, and therefore more instructive, than those commonly found in the works of writers on obstetrics in our own country."

Hirst's Diseases of Women

A Text-Book of Diseases of Women. By BARTON COOKE HIRST, M. D. Octavo of 745 pages, 701 illustrations, many in colors. Cloth, $5.00 net.

SECOND EDITION

As diagnosis and treatment are of the greatest importance in considering diseases of women, particular attention has been devoted to these divisions. The palliative treatment, as well as the radical operation, is fully described, enabling the general practitioner to treat many of his own patients without referring them to a specialist. **Published August, 1905**

Medical Record, New York

"Its merits can be appreciated only by a careful perusal . . Nearly one hundred pages are devoted to technic, this chapter being in some respects superior to the descriptions in other text-books."

Kelly and Noble's Gynecology and Abdominal Surgery

Gynecology and Abdominal Surgery. Edited by HOWARD A. KELLY, M. D., Professor of Gynecology in Johns Hopkins University; and CHARLES P. NOBLE, M.D., formerly Clinical Professor of Gynecology in the Woman's Medical College, Philadelphia. Two imperial octavo volumes of 850 pages each, containing 880 illustrations, mostly original. Per volume : Cloth, $8.00 net ; Half Morocco, $9.50 net. Volume I published May, 1907; Volume II published June, 1908.

WITH 880 ORIGINAL ILLUSTRATIONS BY HERMANN BECKER AND MAX BRÖDEL

In view of the intimate association of gynecology with abdominal surgery the editors have combined these two important subjects in one work. For this reason the work will be doubly valuable, for not only the gynecologist and general practitioner will find it an exhaustive treatise, but the surgeon also will find here the latest technic of the various abdominal operations. It possesses a number of valuable features not to be found in any other publication covering the same fields. It contains a chapter upon the bacteriology and one upon the pathology of gynecology, dealing fully with the scientific basis of gynecology. In no other work can this information, prepared by specialists, be found as separate chapters. There is a large chapter devoted entirely to *medical gynecology*, written especially for the physician engaged in general practice. Heretofore the general practitioner was compelled to search through an entire work in order to obtain the information desired. *Abdominal surgery* proper, as distinct from gynecology, is fully treated, embracing operations upon the stomach, upon the intestines, upon the liver and bile-ducts, upon the pancreas and spleen, upon the kidney, ureter, bladder, and the peritoneum Special attention has been given to *modern technic* The illustrations are the work of *Mr. Hermann Becker* and *Mr Max Brödel*

American Journal of the Medical Sciences

" It is needless to say that the work has been thoroughly done the names of the authors and editors would guarantee this , but much may be said in praise of the method of presentation, and attention may be called to the inclusion of matter not to be found elsewhere."

GET THE BEST — American — THE NEW STANDARD
Illustrated Dictionary
The New (9th) Edition, Reset

The American Illustrated Medical Dictionary. A new and complete dictionary of the terms used in Medicine, Surgery, Dentistry, Pharmacy, Chemistry, Veterinary Science, Nursing, and all kindred branches; with over 100 new and elaborate tables and many handsome illustrations. By W. A. NEWMAN DORLAND, M.D., Editor of "The American Pocket Medical Dictionary." Large octavo, 1179 pages, bound in full flexible leather. Price, $5.00 net; with thumb index, $5.50 net.

A KEY TO MEDICAL LITERATURE

Gives a Maximum Amount of Matter in a Minimum Space

ENTIRELY RESET—2000 NEW WORDS

This edition is not a makeshift revision. The editor and a corps of expert assistants have been working on it for two years. Result—a thoroughly down-to-the-minute dictionary, unequalled for completeness and usefulness by any other medical lexicon published. It meets your wants. It gives you all the *new words*, and in dictionary service *new words* are what you want. Then, it has two-score other features that make it really a *Medical Encyclopedia*.

Published September, 1917

PERSONAL OPINIONS

Howard A. Kelly, M. D.,
Professor of Gynecologic Surgery, Johns Hopkins University, Baltimore.
"Dr. Dorland's dictionary is admirable It is so well gotten up and of such convenient size. No errors have been found in my use of it."

J. Collins Warren, M.D., LL.D., F.R.C.S. (Hon.)
Professor of Surgery, Harvard Medical School.
"I regard it as a valuable aid to my medical literary work. It is very complete and of convenient size to handle comfortably. I use it in preference to any other."

Webster's Diseases of Women

Diseases of Women. By J. Clarence Webster, M. D. (Edin.), F. R. C. P. E., Professor of Gynecology and Obstetrics in Rush Medical College. Octavo of 712 pages, with 372 illustrations. Cloth, $7.00 net.

FOR THE PRACTITIONER

Dr. Webster has written this work *especially for the general practitioner*, discussing the clinical features of the subject in their widest relations to general practice rather than from the standpoint of specialism. The magnificent illustrations, three hundred and seventy-two in number, are nearly all original. Drawn by expert anatomic artists under Dr. Webster's direct supervision, they portray the anatomy of the parts and the steps in the operations with rare clearness and exactness. **Published January, 1907**

Howard A. Kelly, M.D., *Professor of Gynecologic Surgery, Johns Hopkins University.*

" It is undoubtedly one of the best works which has been put on the market within recent years, showing from start to finish Dr. Webster's well-known thoroughness. The illustrations are also of the highest order."

Webster's Obstetrics

A Text-Book of Obstetrics. By J. Clarence Webster, M. D. (Edin.), Professor of Obstetrics and Gynecology in Rush Medical College. Octavo of 767 pages, illustrated. Cloth, $5.00 net. **Published July, 1903**

Medical Record, New York

" The author's remarks on asepsis and antisepsis are admirable, the chapter on eclampsia is full of good material, and . . the book can be cordially recommended as a safe guide."

Kelly *and* Cullen's
Myomata of the Uterus

Myomata of the Uterus. By HOWARD A. KELLY, M. D., Professor of Gynecologic Surgery at Johns Hopkins University; and THOMAS S. CULLEN, M. B., Associate in Gynecology at Johns Hopkins University. Large octavo of about 700 pages, with 388 original illustrations by August Horn and Hermann Becker. Cloth, $7.50 net.

A MASTER WORK
ILLUSTRATED BY AUGUST HORN AND HERMANN BECKER

This monumental work, the fruit of over ten years of untiring labors, will remain for many years the last word upon the subject. Written by those men who have brought, step by step, the operative treatment of uterine myoma to such perfection that the mortality is now less than one per cent., it stands out as the record of greatest achievement of recent times.

The illustrations have been made with wonderful accuracy in detail by Mr. August Horn and Mr. Hermann Becker, whose superb work is so well known that comment is unnecessary. For painstaking accuracy, for attention to every detail, and as an example of the practical results accruing from the association of the operating amphitheater with the pathologic laboratory, this work will stand as an enduring testimonial. **Published May, 1909**

Surgery, Gynecology, and Obstetrics
"It must be considered as the most comprehensive work of the kind yet published. It will always be a mine of wealth to future students."

New York Medical Journal
"Within the covers of this monograph every form, size, variety, and complication of uterine fibroids is discussed. It is a splendid example of the rapid progress of American professional thought."

Bulletin Medical and Chirurgical Faculty of Maryland
"Few medical works in recent years have come to our notice so complete in detail, so well illustrated, so practical, and so far reaching in their teaching to general practitioner, specialist, and student alike."

Penrose's Diseases of Women

Sixth Revised Edition

A Text-Book of Diseases of Women. By CHARLES B. PENROSE, M. D., PH. D., formerly Professor of Gynecology in the University of Pennsylvania; Surgeon to the Gynecean Hospital, Philadelphia. Octavo volume of 550 pages, with 225 fine original illustrations. Cloth $3.75 net. Published March, 1908

ACCURATE

Regularly every year a new edition of this excellent text-book is called for, and it appears to be in as great favor with physicians as with students. Indeed, this book has taken its place as the ideal work for the general practitioner. The author presents the best teaching of modern gynecology, untrammeled by antiquated ideas and methods. In every case the most modern and progressive technique is adopted, and the main points are made clear by excellent illustrations.

Howard A. Kelly, M.D.,
Professor of Gynecologic Surgery, Johns Hopkins University, Baltimore.
"I shall value very highly the copy of Penrose's 'Diseases of Women' received. I have already recommended it to my class as THE BEST book."

Cullen's Uterine Adenomyoma

UTERINE ADENOMYOMA. By THOMAS S. CULLEN, M. D., Associate Professor of Gynecology, Johns Hopkins University. Octavo of 275 pages, with original illustrations by Hermann Becker and August Horn. Cloth, $5.00 net. Published May, 1908

Cullen's Cancer of Uterus

CANCER OF THE UTERUS. By THOMAS S. CULLEN, M. B., Associate Professor of Gynecology, Johns Hopkins University. Large octavo of 693 pages, with over 300 colored and half-tone text-cuts and eleven lithographs. Cloth, $7.50 net; Half Morocco, $8.50 net.
Published 1900

Davis' Obstetric and Gynecologic Nursing

Obstetric and Gynecologic Nursing. By EDWARD P. DAVIS, A. M., M. D., Professor of Obstetrics in the Jefferson Medical College and Philadelphia Polyclinic; Obstetrician and Gynecologist, Philadelphia Hospital. 12mo of 498 pages, illustrated. Buckram $2.00 net.   Published May, 1917

NEW (5th) EDITION

This volume gives a very clear and accurate idea of the manner to meet the conditions arising during obstetric and gynecologic nursing. The fifth edition has been thoroughly revised.

"Not only nurses, but even newly qualified medical men, would learn a great deal by a perusal of this book. It is written in a clear and pleasant style, and is a work we can recommend."—*The Lancet, London.*

American Pocket Dictionary   New (10th) Edition

THE AMERICAN POCKET MEDICAL DICTIONARY. Edited by W. A. NEWMAN DORLAND, A. M., M. D. With 693 pages. Full leather, limp, $1.25 net; patent thumb index, $1.50 net.   September, 1917

James W. Holland, M. D.,
Professor of Chemistry and Toxicology at the Jefferson Medical College, Philadelphia.

"I am struck at once with admiration at the compact size and attractive exterior. I can recommend it to our students without reserve."

Ashton's Obstetrics   Eighth Edition

ESSENTIALS OF OBSTETRICS. By W. EASTERLY ASHTON, M. D., Professor of Gynecology, University of Pennsylvania. Crown octavo, 290 pages, 125 illustrations. Cloth, $1.25 net. *In Saunders' Question-Compend Series.*   Published January, 1917

Galbraith's Four Epochs of Woman's Life   Third Edition

THE FOUR EPOCHS OF WOMAN'S LIFE: A STUDY IN HYGIENE. Maidenhood, Marriage, Maternity, Menopause. By ANNA M. GALBRAITH, M D. With an Introductory Note by JOHN H. MUSSER, M.D . Published March, 1917.   12mo of 296 pages. Cloth, $1.50 net.

Bandler's The Expectant Mother

THE EXPECTANT MOTHER. By SAMUEL WYLLIS BANDLER, M. D., Professor of Diseases of Women, New York Post-Graduate Medical School and Hospital. 12mo of 213 pages, illustrated. Cloth, $1.25 net. Published August, 1916

Montgomery's Care of Gynecologic Cases

CARE OF PATIENTS· Before, During, and After Operation. By E. E. MONTGOMERY, M. D., LL.D., Professor of Gynecology in Jefferson Medical College. 12mo of 149 pages, illustrated. Cloth, $1.25 net. Published December, 1916

Macfarlane's Gynecology for Nurses — Second Edition

A REFERENCE HAND-BOOK OF GYNECOLOGY FOR NURSES. By CATHARINE MACFARLANE, M. D., Gynecologist to the Woman's Hospital of Philadelphia. 16mo of 156 pages, with 70 illustrations. Flexible leather, $1.25 net. Published May, 1913

A. M. Seabrook, M. D., *Woman's Medical College of Philadelphia.*

" It is a most admirable little book, covering in a concise but attractive way the subject from the nurse's standpoint."

Cragin's Gynecology — Eighth Edition

ESSENTIALS OF GYNECOLOGY By EDWIN B. CRAGIN, M. D., Professor of Obstetrics, College of Physicians and Surgeons, New York. Crown octavo, 240 pages, 62 illustrations. Cloth, $1.25 net. *In Saunders' Question-Compend Series.* Published October, 1913

Schäffer and Norris' Gynecology — Saunders' Atlases

ATLAS AND EPITOME OF GYNECOLOGY. By DR. O. SCHAFFER, of Heidelberg. Edited, with additions, by RICHARD C. NORRIS, A. M., M. D., Assistant Professor of Obstetrics, University of Pennsylvania. 155 illustrations, 272 pages. Cloth, $3.50 net. Published 1900

Schäffer and Edgar's Obstetrics

ATLAS AND EPITOME OF OBSTETRIC DIAGNOSIS AND TREATMENT. By DR. O. SCHAFFER, of Heidelberg. *From the Second Revised German Edition.* Edited, with additions, by J. CLIFTON EDGAR, M. D., Professor of Obstetrics and Clinical Midwifery, Cornell University Medical School, N. Y. With 122 colored figures on 56 plates, 38 text-cuts, and 315 pages of text. Cloth, $3.00 net. *In Saunders' Hand-Atlas Series.* Published January, 1902

Schäffer and Webster's Operative Gynecology

Atlas and Epitome of Operative Gynecology. By Dr. O. Schaffer, of Heidelberg. Edited, with additions, by J. Clarence Webster, M. D. (Edin.), F. R. C. P. E., Professor of Obstetrics and Gynecology in Rush Medical College, in affiliation with the University of Chicago. 42 colored lithographic plates, many text-cuts, a number in colors, and 138 pages of text. *In Saunders' Hand-Atlas Series.* Cloth, $3.00 net.

Much patient endeavor has been expended by the author, the artist, and the lithographer in the preparation of the plates for this Atlas. They are based on hundreds of photographs taken from nature, and illustrate most faithfully the various surgical situations. Dr. Schäffer has made a specialty of demonstrating by illustrations. **Published 1904**

Medical Record, New York
" The volume should prove most helpful to students and others in grasping details usually to be acquired only in the amphitheater itself."

De Lee's Obstetrics for Nurses

Obstetrics for Nurses. By Joseph B. De Lee, M. D., Professor of Obstetrics in the Northwestern University Medical School, Chicago; Lecturer in the Nurses' Training Schools of Mercy, Wesley, Provident, Cook County, and Chicago Lying-In Hospitals. 12mo of 550 pages, fully illustrated.

Published July, 1917   Cloth, $2.75 net.

FIFTH EDITION

While Dr. DeLee has written his work especially for nurses, the practitioner will also find it useful and instructive, since the duties of a nurse often devolve upon him in the early years of his practice. The illustrations are nearly all original and represent photographs taken from actual scenes. The text is the result of the author's many years' experience in lecturing to the nurses of five different training schools.

J. Clifton Edgar, M. D.,
Professor of Obstetrics and Clinical Midwifery, Cornell University, New York
" It is far and away the best that has come to my notice, and I shall take great pleasure in recommending it to my nurses, and students as well."

LANE MEDICAL LIBRARY

To avoid fine, this book should be returned on
or before the date last stamped below.

FEB 18 1941

LANE MEDICAL LIBRARY
STANFORD UNIVERSITY
300 PASTEUR DRIVE
PALO ALTO, CALIF.

M151 K26 1918	Keen, W.W. 82487 The treatment of war wounds.	
NAME		DATE DUE
Allen Altman		FEB 13 1941